POVERTY,
ETHNIC IDENTITY,
AND HEALTH CARE

APPLETON-CENTURY-CROFTS / New York
A Publishing Division of Prentice-Hall, Inc.

POVERTY, ETHNIC IDENTITY, AND HEALTH CARE

BONNIE BULLOUGH, R.N., Ph.D.
Assistant Professor of Nursing
University of California, Los Angeles
Los Angeles, California

VERN L. BULLOUGH, Ph.D.
Professor of History
San Fernando Valley State College
Northridge, California;
Lecturer, School of Public Health
University of California, Los Angeles
Los Angeles, California

Library of Congress Catalog Card Number 73–175285

Prentice-Hall International, Inc., London
Prentice-Hall of Australia, Pty. Ltd., Sydney
Prentice-Hall of India Private Limited, New Delhi
Prentice-Hall of Japan, Inc., Tokyo
Prentice-Hall of Southeast Asia (Pte.) Ltd., Singapore

PRINTED IN THE UNITED STATES OF AMERICA 0–8385–7906–X

To
William Henry
and all children who live in poverty

Preface

Though the American health care delivery system has long been in need of reform, its deficiences are only now receiving widespread public scrutiny. This new push for reform has been stimulated by a combination of factors, not the least of which is that our expectations for health care have grown with the medical triumphs of the twentieth century. As medicine has been able to do more we have come to expect more of it. The nature of medical practice has also changed from the individual family doctor or nurse to the team of specialists who have little personal or intimate contact with most of the people they treat or care for. The very impersonality of medical practice tends to lead people to challenge its deficiences more openly. Moreover the rapidly escalating costs of health care in recent years have encouraged feelings of discontent in more segments of society. The discontent is legitimate. In spite of the fact that Americans spend more money on health care than the citizens of any other country that expenditure has not paid off by giving us better health than the rest of the world. The average life expectancy of Americans is lower and the infant and maternal mortality rates are higher than those of many other economically well-developed nations and even some of those which are not particularly prosperous.

The inadequacies of the system are not, however, distributed equally throughout society; the burden tends to fall particularly hard on the poor and on members of the visible minority groups. These are the people this book is about. Their health deficit in relation to the more affluent members of society is a significant factor in the unfavorable statistical picture which emerges when the American system is compared with those of the other highly civilized nations. The result is a national scandal.

The two authors of this book come with a variety of perspectives. One of us is an old nurse and a new sociologist. The other is a medical historian, a civil libertarian, and somewhat of a social critic. That makes us a full committee instead of just a team.

We have tried to bring all of these perspectives to bear on the inadequacies in our health care delivery system. We have tried to avoid glib solutions and to present the problems in all of their complexities. Although we both want to see the enactment of some type of national health insurance we know that this will not solve all of the problems because poverty and discrimination are also implicated as root causes of poor health.

Our concern for this situation dates back to our high school days. The writing we did at that time was produced on smudgy mimeographed underground newsletters which undoubtedly were read only by others who contributed to the same paper. Our first officially published article on discrimination in health care came out in 1952. We have been collecting data and developing the perspective for this book since then, and although we have written several other books in the meantime, this is the one we always wanted to write.

Anyone who uses government documents as we did in this study can only give thanks to the useful services of librarians. For assistance in this and other tasks we would like to specially acknowledge the help of Charlotte Oyer, Frederick Holler, Irene Thorsell, Virginia Sherman, Steven Tash, Margaret Deacon, Ann Waggoner and Helen Bennett, all reference librarians at San Fernando Valley State College. Thanks is also due to Linda Tanz who so carefully typed the manuscript.

Bonnie and Vern Bullough   January 1972

Contents

Preface   vi

Acknowledgment   ix

1.   *THE HEALTH CARE DELIVERY PROBLEM*   1

2.   *IMMIGRANT MINORITY GROUPS*   18

3.   *BLACK AMERICANS*   37

4.   *THE SPANISH-SPEAKING MINORITY GROUPS*   63

5.   *THE NATIVE AMERICANS*   89

6.   *POVERTY AND HUNGER TRANSCEND RACIAL LINES*   109

7.   *MENTAL HEALTH AND MENTAL ILLNESS*   129

8.   *DISCRIMINATION AND SEGREGATION*   147

9.   *IMPROVING HEALTH CARE DELIVERY*   166

Bibliography   199

Index   219

POVERTY,
ETHNIC IDENTITY,
AND HEALTH CARE

The Health Care Delivery Problem

Poverty is an obvious factor in the problem of providing adequate health care. Not so obvious, however, are the difficulties of communicating the health needs of the underprivileged to those in a position to do something about it. A good example of this is the problem of rats, a subject which induced a great deal of laughter when it was introduced in Congress in 1968.[1]

Rats, however, are no laughing matter. Since the beginning of the 20th century it has been known that the fleas which live on infected rats are the common carriers of bubonic plague. Rat populations the world over are carefully watched. The United States has been lucky in that it has never suffered a severe epidemic of the plague, although the bacillus is known to have entered this country in 1900 and to have caused the death of 113 people over a four-year period in San Francisco. Today plague is endemic in the southwestern parts of the United States but the chief animal vectors are squirrels and rabbits, and Americans have continued to be less concerned about rats than most other peoples.

The lack of governmental concern has led to rats' becoming a serious environmental hazard to the poor who inhabit the slums.

This occurs because while it is possible for individual home owners rather easily to rid their property of rats, tenants in large buildings are dependent upon the owners or managers of the buildings. In older buildings even this is not enough because rats have established nests and routes inside the walls, under the flooring, and in the basement, and if one landowner mounts an effective program, the rats simply flee to a neighboring building. To be really effective a rat control program has to involve governmental action on a large scale. Because such programs are usually lacking it has become necessary to give welfare recipients in some of the large cities small supplementary "rat allowances" to enable them to keep their lights burning all night to frighten away the rats.[2]

Such allowances, however, are at best a makeshift solution. The danger that rats pose to children was learned by one of the authors of this book from personal experience. We include it because it exemplifies a type of health care problem which does not touch the affluent members of society and because it emphasizes the communication gap between the rich and the poor. Part of this anecdote is written in the first person because it was taken from notes kept while the author served as a public health nurse in the early 1950s on Chicago's South Side.

In 1953 rats mutilated and killed an infant in an area next to the district in which I was working. In my own district they chewed the hand of a small black newborn infant named William Henry.[3] William's mother and four siblings lived in a dug-out basement under a dilapidated row house. Mrs. Henry had been awakened in the middle of the night by the cries of her baby and found two huge grey rats on top of him. When she snatched him up his hand was a bleeding mass of mangled flesh. She took her baby to Cook County Hospital for emergency care.

Cook County, however, was more than an hour away by bus and in order to get there she borrowed money from her neighbors to take a taxi. Because she was afraid to leave her other four children alone at home she took all of them with her and they spent the night in the emergency room, waiting for the baby to be treated and admitted. Most of William's hand could be saved although he lost the distal portion of three fingers. When William was discharged from the hospital the Health Department was notified. I was sent to visit the family. I found them living in a basement which had probably never been meant to be used as a residence.

Most of the houses in this particular area had been built 60 or 70 years earlier, long before electrical outlets were a standard feature in a home, and when food storage posed serious problems. The basements in these houses had been designed to store food and coal and the original owners probably never thought of these dugouts as a possible residence. It obviously was not a suitable place for five children to live.

> I felt the rats would again attack the infant unless something was done. I called the office of the city housing inspector, met with officials in the urban renewal office, and had long discussions with my own supervisor. In spite of all my efforts, some of which became quite frantic, no public official could be talked into doing anything about the rats, and there seemed to be no other housing available at the level the Henry family could afford.

Rather, it should be said, there was low-income housing available in Chicago at that time, but it was not available to Negroes—even Negroes who were quite well-to-do. The Chicago ghetto had burst the officially imposed boundaries in the years following the 1947 U.S. Supreme Court decision that made restrictive convenants unenforceable. Even with the help of the ever-present block busters the informal pressure against integration in housing or a rapid expansion of the ghetto had kept the "black belt" much too small for the number of people seeking housing. This meant that housing for Negroes rented at about twice the price per room of that available for white families. Inevitably landlords broke up apartments into smaller and smaller units, rented out storage areas, and expected several families to share a bathroom and kitchen.

> Mrs. Henry lived in this ghetto and like many of her neighbors she was on welfare. Her welfare checks were smaller than those of families of comparable size because she had tried to keep the arrival of her new baby a secret. She was convinced that her social worker would cut off her aid entirely if it became known that she had conceived again without finding a stable male breadwinner for the family.
> The house above the Henrys' basement was scheduled to be torn down as a part of a large urban renewal project. The official at the Office of Urban Renewal whom I contacted explained that his department might eventually use its influence to place the

Henrys in public housing since finding other kinds of replacement housing for such a large family on the open market, at a price they could afford, was next to impossible.

The official, however, refused to speed up the process or even let Mrs. Henry know that she had a chance to obtain public housing, because he felt it would be "bad for neighborhood morale." He explained to me that the only way to get "those old mamas off their cans" was to frighten them with the bulldozer. He stated there were not enough public housing units to accomodate all the people who were displaced by urban renewal projects, so that his job of finding replacement housing was much easier if he could convince the people in the buildings which were scheduled to be cleared that they would have to find an apartment for themselves or face the prospect of being in the house when the wrecking crew arrived. Most of the tenants in the buildings which already had been razed had relocated themselves by moving into other slum housing or doubling-up with relatives.

The doubling-up had added to the slum problem by creating the overcrowding which is a major factor in the rapid deterioration of the central city ghetto housing. Not only does such crowding rapidly wear out a building but when large numbers of families use a single facility, such as a kitchen, it is difficult to fix responsibility for keeping the area clean or repaired.

As far as rats were concerned the slum clearance project was a major factor in creating the problem in the first place. This is because the large luxury buildings being built on the cleared land were virtually ratproof. The displaced rats, just as the displaced people, made their way into nearby slum areas. Because of increased concentration, the appetites of the rats soon outstripped the available uncollected garbage supplies and they turned to attacking infants in their cribs.

Several families in the area had built heavy screen cages over their childrens' beds and sometimes at night they would hear rats gnawing on the screens. Mrs. Henry, however, lacked money to buy screens and apparently also had little talent as a carpenter. After the baby came home from the hospital she tried to keep herself awake at night to guard him, but soon a state of chronic exhaustion made this difficult. In a desperate attempt to do something constructive to help her out I begged two half-grown cats from another family I knew and took them to her. Before a week was past the rats had eaten the cats.

Poverty and Ethnic Identity

The Henry family was black and poor. This particular combination of circumstances rendered them relatively powerless to deal with their problem. Affluent Negro families could afford somewhat better housing while poor white families could secure much better housing for the same amount of money. Because the Henrys were poor they had no family doctor and because they were black no South Side emergency room would then treat William.[4] These two factors, poverty and a minority status, are implicated in numerous ways in the present crisis in health care. Although poverty is probably the most important variable because health care is still regarded as a commodity to be purchased on the open market, membership in a low-status minority group adds another dimension to the problem when it comes to achieving good health or obtaining health service. Not only is discrimination present in the delivery of health service but there is also discrimination in the recruitment of health workers. This further adds to the difficulty because the social distance between the worker who is a member of the dominant group and the minority patient often creates a barrier to communication. Moreover, poverty itself is frequently a product of discrimination in education and in hiring so that the variables of poverty and minority status become closely interrelated. In parts of this book poverty and ethnic identity will be separated conceptually but it is important to realize that in the real world the separation is not so easy to make.

Poverty Indexes

In 1965 the Social Security Administration developed an index to measure the economic well-being of families, with the result that poverty could be stated in somewhat more scientific terms. The index took into account such factors as the size and the composition of the family, and whether it lived in an urban or rural setting. For a nonfarm family of four, the poverty level was pegged at approximately $3,335 in 1966 or about three times the minimum amount it was calculated that it would cost to feed them. The dollar income for farm families was slightly lower because it was assumed that farmers had other food resources available to them. Slightly above the poverty level was a second category of "near-poor" families whose income in urban areas was above $3,335 but below $4,345. Calculations were made to adjust the index back to 1959 so that comparisons over a decade were possible, and year-by-year adjustments are made in the index to keep it up-to-date and to allow for changes in the cost of living.

With the use of this index it was estimated that in 1959 there were 38.9 million Americans in some 13.4 million families who were classified as poor. By 1969 the number had fallen to 24.3 million persons in 5 million families.[5] The drop was due to the relatively high employment rates during the decade; but, not surprisingly, the people who left the ranks of the poor were usually young, white healthy adults. This meant that, comparatively, the number of low-income persons who were unskilled, chronically ill, or were members of minority groups increased proportionately. Large numbers of those classified as poor were under 18 or over 64. The older people are more likely to live alone and the children are more likely to be members of families larger than the United States average. Nearly half of the family units which were classified at or below the poverty line were headed by a woman.[6] This indicates that most of the people who are classified as poor would not be helped by a simple expansion of our economy because they tend to be unavailable for better-paying work either because of their age, family responsibilities, poor health, lack of ability, or the barriers of discrimination.

In 1959 nonwhite families made up about one-fourth of the families classified as poor, but at latest count they made up approximately one-third. Though the majority of poor and near-poor are still white (including Appalachian residents, Mexican-Americans, and some Puerto Ricans), members of nonwhite minority groups, particularly Negroes and Indians, are overrepresented among the ranks of the poor. Because of the current increase in unemployment the number of people who fall below the poverty line has again increased to 25.5 million, so that the problem of poverty is still very much with us and will remain until we face up to the problem of dealing with it.[7]

Socioeconomic Status and Health

Compounding poverty and making it more difficult to overcome is the fact that people with low incomes are more likely to suffer from illnesses than those whose income is higher. In a recent nationwide survey the health needs and problems of American families were studied. It was found that 44 percent of the more affluent families had a sick family member at the time of the survey, while 65 percent of the ghetto black families and 75 percent of the Appalachian white families reported a family member suffering from a current illness. A similar pattern emerged when people were asked if there was someone in the family who had taken sick within the last month. One-third of the total number of respondents reported someone had become ill in the month, but approximately one-half of the poverty families so reported.[8]

Differences in morbidity also are associated with ethnic status. The kinds of illnesses that Negroes are more likely to have are often different from those which afflict whites. For instance, the incidence of cardiovascular diseases, untreated cancer, tuberculosis, pneumonia, and diabetes is especially high among blacks. [9] Mexican-Americans are more likely to suffer from pneumonia than Anglos,[10] and Indians have particularly high rates of tuberculosis, dysentery, pneumonia,[11] and suicide.[12]

In spite of some of the mythology about the stress and strain of being rich, the high-powered executive is much less likely to end up in a mental hospital than the unemployed black man. The link between low socioeconomic status and mental illness was first noted by the early sociologists of the Chicago school who found that hospitalized mental patients were more likely to come from certain neighborhoods.[13] Generations of researchers have now explored this correlation of socioeconomic status and mental health in depth. Most everyone agrees that the key to cure is early treatment. Although health care professionals argue that neuroses and psychoses are different, somehow people with adequate incomes tend to be diagnosed early as neurotic and are treated so that they can continue to function in society. Individuals whose incomes are lower are seldom treated early, and when they are finally diagnosed they are classified as psychotic and are more likely to end up in large state mental hospitals.[14]

Illnesses of the poor also tend to be more serious, so that death or disability are more likely to follow than in upper-income groups. Mortality rates for nonwhites and people whose socioeconomic status are low are correspondingly higher. In 1965 the life expectancy for the newborn white American, regardless of economic background, was 70.2 years; for the newborn nonwhite it was 63.6.[15] This means that having the good fortune to be born white gives one an extra seven years of life. The delivery of the infant is also more perilous for the nonwhite mother; her risk of death at delivery is three times that of a white mother, with the maternal mortality rate in 1966 of 72.4 per 100,000 live births for nonwhites as compared to 20.2 for white mothers.[16] This high death rate can be related to many factors, including inadequate prenatal care, fewer hospital deliveries, less contact with specialists, less adequate nutrition, and the poor general health of the average nonwhite mother.[17]

It is not the maternal mortality rates but the infant rates that have received the greatest public attention in recent years. Since infant death rates have been regarded as an index to the general well-being of a society, United States has for the past 50 years paid considerable attention to them. In 1950 we had achieved an infant mortality rate of 29.2 per 1,000 live births and we were justly proud because it represented a great decline from the 1900 rate of 100 and the 1935 rate of 55.7. Our infant mortality rate in 1950 was the sixth lowest in the world,[18] but this marked a sort of plateau. Although the rate has continued to decline, comparatively speaking the United States looks worse as one by one the advanced nations of the world have passed us up. By 1963 we had fallen to fourteenth place, with a rate of 25.2 deaths per 1,000 live births. In 1969 our infant mortality rate was 20.8 which gave us a rank order of sixteenth place. Iceland, the leader, had a rate of 11.7.[19] Several Eastern European countries which still have mortality rates higher than ours have shown a rapid rate of improvement, and if the present trend continues they will soon pass us up. Table 1 shows the rank ordering of the major countries.

TABLE 1. Infant Mortality Rates*

	1969	1963	1953
Iceland	11.7	17.0	19.0
Sweden	13.0**	15.4	18.7
Netherlands	13.2	15.8	23.7
Norway	13.7**	16.9	22.0
Finland	13.9	18.2	34.2
Denmark	14.8	19.1	27.2
Japan	15.3	23.2	48.9
Switzerland	15.4	20.5	29.8
France	16.4	25.4	41.9
Luxembourg	16.7	28.6	42.3
Australia	17.8**	19.5	23.3
Ukrainian SSR	18.4	24.3	63.0
United Kingdom (England, Wales, Scotland & Northern Ireland)	18.6	21.8	27.6
New Zealand	18.7**	19.6	25.7
Taiwan (Nationalist China)	19.1	26.4	33.7
East Germany	20.0	31.4	53.5
Ireland	20.6	26.6	39.4
Singapore	20.7	27.9	67.1
United States	20.8	25.2	27.8

* Deaths of infants under one year of age per 1,000 live births.
** Latest available figures were from 1968.

From the United Nations, Statistical Office, Statistical Yearbook, 1969.
(New York: United Nations Publishing Service, 1970) pp. 99-101.

The question that must be asked is: Why the decline in our position relative to other countries? Since we have by far the largest gross national product the mortality figures cannot be attributed to our lack of economic development. Our higher infant mortality rate is not due to lack of medical knowledge, since our medical expertise and research capabilities are second to none. Rather it seems obvious that our drop in comparative position is due to the unequal distribution of materials, resources, and health care as well as to our system of priorities that places emphasis upon more dramatic types of health services, such as heart transplants, rather than the actual application of knowledge which is already at hand. Thus the mortality rate for nonwhite infants in 1970 was 31.4 per 1,000 live births while the rate for white infants was 17.4; the black child was almost twice as likely to die as his white counterpart.[20] The figures are comparable when income alone is used as a variable.

An examination of Table 1 will indicate that those countries which have passed up the United States have several things in common. They tend to be countries with fairly homogenous population, no steep differences in income levels, and they have some system of national health insurance which delivers adequate health care to all of the people, not just those who can buy it on the open market. In the United States, in spite of the fact that illness is likely both to be more common and to lead to death and disability among the poor, medical care for low-income people is inferior in both quality and quantity to that received by the more well-to-do members of society.

During the fiscal year ending in June 1967, it was calculated that the average American saw a physician 4.3 times (including home, office, and hospital visits). People with family incomes of less than $5,000 and nonwhites as a group averaged 3.1 visits.[21] One reason for the disparity is the fact that practicing physicians are sparse in poor residential areas. For example, the South Health District of Los Angeles (which includes the area where the Watts riot took place) in 1965 contained 65 physicians, or a ratio of 45 physicians per 100,000 population. The nearby Southeast district had an even lower ratio of 38 doctors per 100,000 population. The total Los Angeles County ratio was 127 physicians per 100,000 persons—or about three times the number found in the poorer areas.[22] A shortage of doctors in the areas of the highest illness is undoubtedly due in part to the fact that most physicians find it more profitable to practice in affluent neighborhoods, but the long tradition of discrimination against minority candidates in medicine and the related health professions cannot be overlooked as an important factor in the situation.

Quite obviously persons below the poverty line cannot usually afford the services of a private physician in any case, so that hospital out-patient facilities and emergency rooms serve as the basic source of essential medical care for them. Unfortunately, as the cost of medical services has escalated, private hospitals have of necessity curtailed their charity work. Even hospitals with medical school ties have substituted "teaching beds" for "charity beds," and this has led to further discrimination. Interns and residents are attracted to those institutions which best guarantee them interesting and challenging cases with which to perfect their skills. Inevitably, indigent patients with unusual illnesses can be treated free by a resident or intern and by highly specialized teachers but if the poor man's diagnosis is less "interesting" he has little chance of care in a private hospital.

The result has been an increase in the patient load of the tax-supported hospitals, often without a corresponding expansion of facilities or staff. The physician in the typical county hospital who diagnoses and treats the patient is at best a resident, and not infrequently he is a medical student or an intern. Since even the resident is supposedly still in training, we have a health care system in which poor people are reduced to the status of "clinical material" so that young physicians can gain experience in order later to treat their own private patients.[23]

Medical care for the poor is also fragmented care. Preventive health care—including immunizations, prenatal care, and well-baby care—is not infrequently furnished to the public in clinics run by health departments, but usually these clinics do not treat persons who are ill. This means that when the patient does go to the hospital because he is sick, there is no medical record that can be used to assist in diagnosing his illness or to understand his background. All of the personnel at the institution are strangers to him. If he suffers from chronic or recurrent illnesses he may become well-acquainted with the nursing personnel, but rotating interns move as often as every month from one clinical area to another. Under these conditions the close "doctor-patient relationship" so valued by American medicine becomes little more than a myth. Some poor people accept this system without complaint because they have no choice, but some patients withdraw from treatment. As one 73-year-old patient explained to her social worker:

> I ain't going back 'cause the last time I was there they had twelve boy doctors looking at this leg. I ain't no guinea pig.[24]

Others are more willing to accept the system but still find it impossible, as did a mother of four, who reported:

> I went there at 9:00 like they said. About 12:30 I saw the doctor and he said I was in the wrong clinic. I went to the other clinic and waited until 2:00 and there were still people in front of

me. The kids get out of school at 2:30 so I had to leave. No, I don't blame them; that's just the way it is if you're poor.[25]

Changing Nature of Medical Care

The poor have always been part of the American scene, but their health care problems have become much more serious in the last few decades. One of the reasons for the growing seriousness of the problem is the rapid, almost revolutionary, changes which have taken place in medicine. Since the turn of the century the nature of medicine has changed from being more or less custodial to materially assisting in the cure of the patient. During the same period hospitals changed from eleemosynary institutions run by religious or charitable bodies to centers of scientific medicine, and some of them have even become profit-making institutions.

Such changes have also modified the relationship of the doctor to the patient. At the turn of the century doctors had a one-to-one relationship with their patient, and it was not unusual for the local physician to vary his fees according to the economic circumstances of his patients. Moreover, the qualifications for becoming a physician were not particularly arduous or time-consuming and the doctor's income was not proportionately much different from that of the grocer or the other small businessman. This meant that physicians were likely to live in all parts of the city, although the wealthier ones undoubtedly lived in the higher-income areas since their wealth came from serving upper-income patients. Childbirth was most likely to take place under the supervision of the midwife, and in the care of the critically ill the nurse was as important as the physician. Slum dwellers or poor people in the city never saw a doctor until they were seriously ill, and then they were likely to depend upon a charity hospital for care. In fact, hospitals were regarded as places for poor patients to go, and they were often attached to a medical school or had a number of volunteer physicians who donated their services. Well-to-do people were treated in their own homes under the supervision of a private-duty nurse.

During the course of the 20th century more and more of the medical tasks became institutionalized. Childbirth, which previously had been centered in the home, moved into the hospital. Developments in anesthesia, in obstetrical surgery, in special equipment and better aseptic techniques, as well as the changing nature of the American family, all contributed to the move. So did the invention of the incubator as well as other devices for infant care that could only be found in the hospitals. Scientific breakthroughs of the 19th and 20th centuries made operative wounds less prone to become infected, and hundreds of new surgical techniques were developed allowing the surgeon to operate on the chest, brain, heart, and other parts of the body that earlier would not have been probed. In addition to the improvements in asepsis and anesthesia the perfection of transfusion aided the development of surgery. With the development of the rapid frozen-section method, surgery also became a diagnostic tool. The invention of x-ray equipment, the electroencephalograph, radioactive-isotopes techniques, and numerous other tools for treatment and diagnosis led to greater and greater concentration of patients in the hospitals in order to make better use of the investment required to operate such equipment. Further encouraging the growth of hospitals was the development of health insurance, which was primarily an innovation born during the depression of the 1930s. Health insurance in the United States usually only paid for claims incurred during hospitalization, and many diagnostic and minor surgical procedures that could have been performed in the doctor's office were transferred to the hospital.

Education for physicians was upgraded; the length of training was increased while proportionately the number of doctors in the population was deliberately decreased, and physicians' income grew rapidly. Most of the changes in the nature of training were initiated by the American Medical Association in a conscious effort to upgrade both medical services and the income of individual practitioners. As part of the effort medical schools themselves changed. Fewer and fewer medical schools utilized the county hospitals as the main source of "guinea pig" patients, and instead moved on to the university campus where "teaching beds" replaced charity beds. Interns and residents found a growing variety of hospitals that wanted their services, and in order to compete county hospitals had to pay for their medical staff.

Developments in medicine coincided with similar changes in nursing. In the years following World War II, the nature of the hospital training school changed as more and more nurses went to collegiate or community-college schools of nursing. In the period before World War II the vast majority of hospitals had been run by student nurses who received little more than their board, room, and "education" for their work. With the upgrading of nursing schools, hospitals were no longer able to recruit a supply of underpaid student laborers, and increasingly professional staffs replaced student nurses. This meant that hospitals had to pay for their staffs, and the cost of hospitalization rose accordingly.

These and other changes in medicine and nursing led to a growing crisis in medical care. Add to them the disabilities inherent in a discriminatory system and the crisis reaches epidemic proportions. Unfortunately the United States has never developed any comprehensive plan to deal with the medical crisis. In fact, the whole history of medical care of the poor in this country indicates that there has not ever been any well-thought-out plan but rather health programs have taken the path of least resistance. In most cases such programs did not take into account the welfare of the poor patients as a prime consideration. Even the public health measures in the United States have most often been instituted in those areas which concern middle- and upper-class Americans and not to satisfy the health needs of the poor. The fact that American public health has concentrated in the area either of the least resistance or that which is most popular to middle- and upper-income groups is evident from the emphasis given to sanitation, immunization, and epidemiology.

Once the contagious nature of certain diseases was established by such men as Louis Pasteur and Robert Koch, it was relatively easy to convince citizens and taxpayers to support wide-scale sanitation and immunization efforts if only because it was obvious that infectious diseases spread to all segments of society. Though the poor benefited greatly from such programs, it was the fact that immunizing the poor child cut down the spread of disease to the middle-class child which made such measures so politically potent. The middle-class bias in control of contagious disease is perhaps nowhere more evident that in the types of disease which public health officials worked the hardest to control. Poliomyelitis is a good case in point because it was probably more likely to leave its crippling aftereffects in the richer areas than the poor. This was because in the crowded urban slums the disease was quickly passed around so that children had frequent exposures while they were young and often developed mild cases which gave lasting immunity without the crippling aftereffects. Middle- and upper-class children who were more protected tended to contract the disease at a later age and were often likely to be permanently crippled—as was so dramatically demonstrated by the case of President Franklin D. Roosevelt. Following President Roosevelt's lead, money was raised by the March of Dimes to finance a vigorous research program as well as to buy equipment and give treatment to poliomyelitis victims. Ultimately the program led to the Salk and indirectly to the Sabin vaccines. Tuberculosis research and therapy, on the other hand, received very little public support—although it was a far more dangerous disease in that it killed 33,633 people in 1950 compared to poliomyelitis, which killed 1,686. Tuberculosis, however, was a disease which mainly stayed in the slums—where it killed rather than gave immunity.[26] Tuberculosis today is still common among the less affluent minority groups such as Indians, Mexican-Americans, and Negroes, but it is not very common among affluent whites.

This is not to say that the public health movement has focused on certain diseases or problems out of any malicious neglect, but simply that funds and resources are limited, the problems are vast, and it is politically feasible to concentrate on some things to the exclusion of others. When poor people are recipients of programs designed specifically for the poor, the emphasis is usually either consciously or unconsciously in a noncontroversial area such as the care of infants, pregnant mothers, or crippled children. In many cases these programs, most of which were established in the 1930s, took over existing charitable enterprises which had already focused public attention on the problem. It was also easy for public health programs to enter into areas where public institutions already existed, such as the school health program. To set up brand new institutions to deal with health problems was much more difficult to accomplish.

The result is that medical care for the poor today is very spotty. Pregnant mothers and well babies receive the most attention, school children are the focus of some programs, and with the advent of Medicare, senior citizens also receive some care. People with rare diseases receive outstanding care because they are of interest to medical schools or to hospital staffs which have teaching beds at their disposal. For the rest, however, even with Medicare and Medicaid, present medical care is inadequate. The factors present in the current crisis in health care will receive somewhat more detailed analysis in this book, but obviously the answer to the crisis involves a rethinking of our whole health care delivery system.

Notes

1. *The Congressional Record* for 1968 and 1969 includes several discussions on rats. Senate Bill 576 was introduced in January 1969 to extend rat control programs and Senator Jacob Javits had to emphasize in his speech that rat control was no laughing matter.
2. H. Jack Geiger, "The Endlessly Revolving Door," *American Journal of Nursing* (November 1969), pp. 2435-2445.
3. This is a fictitious name to protect William's privacy, although considering the opportunities available to a slum child of that time it is doubtful that he or many of his peers would have become a health professional, a sociologist, or other readers of books such as this one. One of the characteristics of our present problem in health care delivery is that the victims of the inequities of the system are also cut off from the educational opportunities that would have allowed them to read the scholarly literature about their problems.
4. It should be noted that legislation passed in recent years would make illegal the open exclusion of William from emergency care because he was black. Even today, however, he would face more subtle kinds of economic and racial discrimination and in most cases he would still have to be taken to a county or other such hospital for treatment.
5. Mollie Orshansky, "The Poverty Roster," *Sources* (Chicago: The Blue Cross Association, 1968), pp. 4-19.; U.S. Bureau of Census, Current Population Reports, P-60, No. 76, "24 Million Americans—Poverty in the United States-1969" (Washington D.C.: U.S. Government Printing Office, 1970), pp. 1-5.
6. Orshansky, *op. cit.*
7. United States Bureau of the Census, *Current Population Reports* Series P-60, No. 70, "Consumer Income." (Washington, D. C.: U.S. Government Printing Office, 1971), p. 1.
8. Louis Harris, "How the Poor View Their Health," *Sources*, p. 25.
9. Mark Lepper, Joyce Lashof, Monroe Lerner, Jeremiah German, and Samuel L. Angeleman, "Approaches to Meeting Health Needs of Large Poverty Populations," *American Journal of Public Health*, 57 (July 1967), pp. 153-57.
10. A. Taher Moustafa and Gertrude Weiss, *Health Status and Practices of Mexican Americans*, Advance Report II, Mexican-American Study Project (University of California, Los Angeles, School of Public Health, 1968).

11. Senator and Mrs. Fred L. Harris, "Indian Health," *Sources,* p. 38.
12. *Suicide Among the American Indians: Two Workshops, Aberdeen, South Dakota, 1967, Lewistown, Montana, November, 1967,* U.S. Dept. of Health, Education, and Welfare, Public Health Service Publication No. 1903 (Washington, D.C.: U.S. Government Printing Office, 1969).
13. Robert E. L. Faris and H. Warren Dunham, *Mental Disorders in Urban Areas* (Chicago: University of Chicago Press, 1939).
14. Jerome K. Meyers, Lee L. Bean, and Max P. Pepper, "Social Class and Psychiatric Disorders: A Ten Year Follow Up," *Journal of Health and Human Behavior,* 6 (Summer 1965), pp. 74-78.
15. U.S. Department of Health, Education, and Welfare, Human Investment Programs: *Delivery of Health Services for the Poor,* December 1967 (Washington, D.C.: U.S. Government Printing Office, 1967), p. 40.
16. United States Department of Health, Education, and Welfare, Health Service, *Vital Statistics of the United States,* vol. II, *Mortality* (Washington, D.C.: U.S. Government Printing Office, 1968), pp. 1-41.
17. Sam Shapiro, Edward R. Schlesinger, and Robert E. L. Nesbitt, Jr., *Infant, Perinatal, Maternal, and Childhood Mortality in the United States* (Cambridge: Harvard University Press, 1968).
18. *Ibid.,* p. 116
19. United Nations, Statistical Office, *Statistical Yearbook, 1969* (New York: United Nations Publishing Service, 1970), pp. 99-101.
20. United States Department of Health, Education, and Welfare, *Monthly Vital Statistics Report,* Provisional Statistics, "Annual Summary for the United States, 1970: Births, Deaths, Marriages and Divorces," (Washington, D.C.: U.S. Government Printing Office), p. 5.
21. United States Department of Health, Education, and Welfare, "Volume of Physician Visits, United States, July, 1966–June, 1967," *Vital and Health Statistics* (National Center for Health Statistics, Series 10, No. 49), p. 21.
22. Milton I. Roemer, "Health Resources and Services in the Watts Area of Los Angeles," *California's Health* (February-March 1966), pp. 123-143.
23. Raymond S. Duff and August B. Hollingshead, *Sickness and Society* (New York: Harper & Row, 1968).
24. Alonzo Yerby, "Improving Care for the Disadvantaged," *American Journal of Nursing,* 68 (May 1968), p. 1044.
25. *Ibid.*
26. Ozzie G. Simmons, "Implications of Social Class for Public Health," in *A Sociological Framework for Patient Care,* edited by Jeannette R. Folta and Edith S. Deck (New York: John Wiley, 1966).

2

Immigrant Minority Groups

Technically a minority is any racial, religious, occupational, or other group constituting less than a numerical majority of the population. All of us belong to various kinds of minorities in this sense. In a more real sense, however, a minority group needs protection and encouragement from the overpowering majority which controls the government since they are often looked down upon because of racial, religious, or even economic reasons. The constitution in fact was designed to protect such minorities by its due process and equal protection clause. Nevertheless, in spite of the constitutional guarantees, minorities have traditionally suffered all kinds of discrimination, even ostracism, in the United States.

In the early history of this country minority status was based mostly upon religion, but in the 19th century it came to be identified with place of national origin as well as religion; in the 20th century, racial and economic factors have more often been the basis for designation as a minority. Every high-school student knows that America has been made up by different groups of immigrants, but it is not always so evident that these immigrants were themselves for a time minority group members, and had many of the same problems as today's minority group members. Emigration was a traumatic experience. It took people out of their traditional environments and replanted them in strange settings, among strange people, and even stranger customs. Old modes of behavior were no longer adequate to meet the new and quite different problems of life. The responses of the newly arrived prospective citizen were not easy or automatic, for emigration had changed the underlying nature of the social structure to which he had been accustomed and neither the complex of institutions nor the societal patterns which formerly guided him were present.

Though some immigrants became rapidly assimilated into the culture of the new country, most of them tried to find people with like ways and customs, settling down together, fearful almost that if they did not retain at least some of the old ways, they themselves would be lost. In the long run this in-group identification of the members of minorities has been both a strength and a weakness for our society. The competing minority groups consciously or unconsciously helped us to achieve our own particular type of pluralistic democracy because the diversity of groups tended to prevent any one faction from achieving a monopoly of power. Even the basic constitutional guarantee of freedom of religion was due in part to the fact that Americans could not agree upon one single religion. On the other hand, ethnic status—based upon religious, national, or racial identity—has also been used as a basis for exploitation and conflict.

Usually as the members of the minority group achieved a measure of power and economic success, they were all too willing to discriminate against the newer minority groups, denying them access to the more pleasant neighborhoods, the better jobs, an adequate education, and even health care. Inevitably this discrimination led to conflict because the deprived groups had imbibed too much of the American dream to be contented with their second-class status, and they too struggled for their share of the good life. In part the history of the United States for the past 100 years has been the history of successive minority groups attempting to move up in American society, and the reaction of the older established groups in opposing them.

Although in many ways the American experience is unique, this is not the only country with minority groups based on ethnic identity. In Europe, minority ethnic populations have been created many times by changing national boundaries. With each new conquest indigenous peoples in the conquered territories have had to adjust to new national identities and have often been pressured to adopt the dominant culture of their new nation. In some disputed areas these changes in national identity have occurred with painful regularity. Alsace-Lorraine has been French, German, French, German, and French in the past century. Poland, which was part of Russia until the end of World War I, found its boundaries moved westward after World War II, taking in areas which had been German, and it lost much of its eastern territory to Russia. There are German-speaking minorities in northern Italy, and Italian-speaking groups in Yugoslavia; Hungarian-speaking groups in Roumania; and the list could go on. Europe has also seen mass migrations of people such as the French-speaking Huguenots into Prussia during the 17th century. Not all minority groups respond to their minority status in the same way. Louis Wirth, a pioneering investigator into minority group problems, proposed a four-fold classification of minority groups based upon their dominant aims: (1) pluralistic, (2) assimilationist, (3) secessionist, and (4) militant. A minority group with a pluralistic aim "seeks toleration for its differences on the part of the dominant group," while an assimilationist minority "craves the fullest opportunity for participation in the life of the larger society." Secessionists, on the other hand, want "to achieve political as well as cultural independence from the dominant group," while a militant minority sets its sights on "domination over others."[1]

In an earlier era before nationalism became such a potent force, most European minority groups were pluralistic in their aims, content with retaining their own language and religion but not particularly vigorous in trying to change their situation. With time, pluralism often led to assimilation as the minority groups accepted the culture of the nation which had conquered them. One of the most notable examples was the city of Strasbourg in France, which until its seizure by the French in 1681 had been German-speaking and Protestant but over a period of time became French-speaking and Catholic. With the rise of nationalism, which gathered tremendous strength in the 19th century, many minority groups became more militant and sought domination by their group over others as the Germans and Hungarians did in the Austro-Hungarian Empire before World War I while some groups sought self-identity as did the Serbs, the Croats, the Roumanians, and others who felt themselves subjugated. There are a few minorities, such as the Basques in Spain and France, who have maintained their identity for thousands of years.

Aiding the growth of nationalism was the expansionist policies of the European imperialistic countries, notably England, France, and Spain. Many of the conquered peoples had never thought of themselves as national groups but their common resentment against conquering powers often led to the growth of such feelings. This has created all kinds of problems in today's world, although in some areas the problem is greater than in other areas because of the nature of European penetration. In many of the conquered lands the imperialist powers were content with economic exploitation and they never became an important part of the culture of the conquered peoples. In some areas, however, the Europeans sent out permanent settlers, reducing the indigenous people to a minority status. This occurred with the Indians in the Americas, the Maoris of New Zealand, the Bushmen of Australia, and the native Hawaiians.

At first the European settlers in these areas were themselves minorities, but they were able to dominate the indigenous people because of their superior technology and ultimately because of their greater numbers. In those areas where the indigenous peoples were more numerous, and where immigration was not so great, as in South Africa and Rhodesia, the Europeans have managed to retain dominance through their greater fire power and political sophistication. In the Republic of South Africa, for example, the white Afrikaners of Dutch descent and the other whites of English origin number only two million in a nation of some 17.5 million people. There are an additional half million Indians, and a half million "colored" whose racial origins are mixed, but outnumbering all of them are the millions of black Africans. Though numerically the black Africans are dominant, real power is held by the white Africans who segregate and exploit the natives, and to a lesser extent the colored and Indian populations. A similar situation is developing in Rhodesia.

American Minority Groups

The United States differs from South Africa in that the immigrants vastly outnumber the indigenous inhabitants. Only the Indians and the Spaniards of the Southwest became minorities by conquest of their homeland. The other American minorities to which all the rest of us belong were willing or unwilling immigrants. The most unwilling to come were the slaves who were brought here and exploited by the European settlers. Other groups of immigrants might also have been reluctant to come, including some of the convicts transported to Georgia or the Chinese imported to build the railroads, but most others came willingly. It could be expected that the willing immigrants would feel more open to assimilation than conquered peoples, and this in fact seems to have been the case. It should be emphasized, however, that many of the Europeans and Asians who came to this country did not intend to stay and settle. Instead they were sojourners who planned to accumulate some wealth and return to their homelands, and in point of fact large numbers of them did return—although not always with the wealth they had dreamed of taking back. Although the statistics describing emigration rates from the United States are not as complete as those describing immigration in the 19th century, early 20th century figures indicate that the emigration rate from United States was not insignificant. In the eight-year period ending in 1915, for example, there were approximately eight million immigrants, but there were four million people who left the country.[2] It has been estimated that about 30 percent of the American immigrants who entered the country between 1821 and 1924 eventually returned to their homeland.[3] It would seem that these sojourners would cling more to the old-country customs than people who were planning to stay permanently, and this had an influence upon the immigrant communities. Moreover, there were probably many millions of others who intended to return to their homeland but because of various circumstances never made it. Nevertheless, the goal of returning to the fatherland undoubtedly encouraged many of them to keep alive their old culture, thus slowing down the rate of assimilation and increasing the generation gap between them and their American-born children.

Adding to the gap between immigrant groups and other Americans was the fact that the homeland of immigrants differed from one era to another. During the colonial period most of the immigrants were from the British Isles, with the largest single identity being Scotch Irish. The Scotch Irish had been relocated in Ireland from the Scottish lowlands during the 17th century, but discontented with an unfavorable land tenure system, they came to the American colonies in increasing numbers during the 18th century, and settled along the frontier. During this same period, there were also a large number of German-speaking settlers from a variety of German states and the German cantons of Switzerland, as well as some Dutch, Swedish, and French Huguenot settlers.[4] Even in this early stage in the settlement of the colonies the tendency for the various groups to form ethnic enclaves could be noted. One of the most striking examples of this separatism took place in Pennsylvania, where the Scotch Irish and German communities grew up along side each other.[5] The continuation of separate ethnic communities is still obvious in Pennsylvania, particularly among the Old Order Amish and other Mennonites who have managed still to cling to many of the customs of the 18th century.

Refugees from the French Revolution swelled the number of immigrants at the end of the 18th century, but it was not until the 19th century that large-scale migration to this country occurred. The first wave followed in the aftermath of the Napoleonic Wars, and there were increases during each successive decade until the 1850s when more than two million Europeans migrated to this country. Although every country in Europe contributed to this outward flow, the majority of immigrants were from the northern and western parts of Europe. The reasons for setting out for America varied. There was a rapid expansion of population in Europe during the period, putting a premium upon land, and increasing numbers of people had heard of the opportunities available in America. Political discontent played a role, as evidenced by the German migration following the failure of the Revolution of 1848, as did religion (witness the converts to the Mormon Church), but the most important motive was an economic one as Europeans sought land, jobs, and a better life. Great national tragedies also played a part in the displacement of populations. The potato blight hit Ireland's main food crop between 1845 and 1849, causing widespread famine and driving many of the survivors to seek new homes and opportunities in America.

The 19th-century newcomer was different from his 18th-century counterpart in the area of settlement. Most 18th-century immigrants had headed for the undeveloped frontier where land was available while the 19th-century immigrants, with a number of exceptions, settled first in the cities—where they sought employment in the developing industries. The newly arrived people moved into the rapidly growing cities' low-rent areas (slum is the term we now use) usually located in and around the business or factory district of the city as the more well-to-do residents had moved farther out. Adjustment to the new world and to new conditions was never easy. Affluent or successful people seldom emigrated to America, so those who did leave home tended to have meager resources, and what little money they did have was used on transportation to the new land. In fact this was one of the reasons these people so often settled in the city rather than the countryside in the 19th and 20th centuries; many of them lacked the resources to go much farther.

Strangers in the immediate world around them, the immigrants fought the loneliness of their condition and created a variety of formal and informal institutions to help them adjust. Usually they settled in the same neighborhood as their former countrymen. In the process they created Germantowns, New Irelands, or Little Polands. Eventually as these settlers became successful some of them were able to move out into more comfortable neighborhoods. The old ethnic neighborhood was then taken over by new immigrants who, like their predecessors, were attracted by the cheap rents and central location. As the changeover took place the new arrivals filtered into the district, occupying house after house as it became vacant until the whole character of a Germantown had changed to a Little Italy or an Irish enclave had given way to a Russian Jewish ghetto. This challenge to the old settled groups by the new was often associated with hostility and conflict.

The immigrants were also exploited. Sometimes this exploitation was by individuals of the same ethnic group whose experience or facility with English enabled them to deal with the more established Americans. Often, however, the manipulation was by outsiders who had little sympathy with or understanding of the new immigrant group, but could use their naiveté, poverty, and lack of English language skills to exploit them. Unfortunately, the very tendency of the immigrant to "ghettoize" himself made him more exploitable. The land near the center of the city might eventually have great value, but only in terms of the land and not for the existing structure. Inevitably the existing housing tended to become dilapidated, and essential repairs were neglected as the owners waited for their land to appreciate. The newcomers lacked the economic or political power to demand improvements. Moreover, the fact that they were segregated made it possible to neglect essential services in their areas without inconveniencing other citizens, so that municipal services—such as garbage collection, street repairs, and police protection—were inferior to those supplied the residents of the newer sections of the city.[6] Schooling for the children of the new immigrants was inferior to that given to pupils whose parents lived in the more affluent sections of the city; buildings were older, staffs smaller, and the children left school at an earlier age than did children who came from families who were higher on the socioeconomic ladder.[7]

The tendency of the new immigrants to form enclaves based on ethnic identity also made it possible for other Americans to accuse them of "clannishness" and to argue that immigrants lived in squalor because they liked it that way. Inevitably when members of the groups did accumulate enough capital to buy homes or rent more comfortable quarters, the "racist" justifications for their earlier exploitation gave them a negative image which worked to exclude them from the outer sections of the city by informal pressures, agreement, and even laws. Irish immigrants in particular were targets for discriminatory action during the mid-19th century because they were the first large group of Catholics to come to this country and many of them had arrived in the most abject poverty. Though America had been founded by religious refugees, most of them were Protestants who had built-in fears of "popery" which the large influx of Irish (and to a lesser extent German) Catholics aroused to fever pitch. Even in the colonial period many of the colonies had charged the captain of ships who brought Catholic immigrants an extra head tax.[8]

In spite of the prejudice against them, the Irish were eventually able to make their way into better-paying jobs in the building trades, as policemen, or as minor political officials. Their paychecks became their weapons against discrimination and they gradually moved out of the central city slum areas. The ingrained nature of the prejudice against them, however, was probably not fully eradicated until John F. Kennedy, an Irishman and a Catholic, was elected President of the United States, thus following in the footsteps of Dwight David Eisenhower, who was of German background. Spiro T. Agnew also becomes a symbolic breakthrough for the more recent Greek immigrants.

As the Irish moved out of the central city slum areas, they were replaced by newer groups: the Italians, Hungarians, Bohemians, Poles, Russians, and new waves of Germans, Swedes, and others. Again, the new immigrants—employed in the most menial and low-paying jobs—were able only to rent quarters in the most deteriorated sections of the city. Few of the immigrants from eastern and southern Europe were Protestants or even Catholics. Large numbers were either Orthodox Christians or Jews, so that their religious identity proved an additional source of prejudice from both Protestant and Catholic Americans.

Those people most accustomed to minority status were the Jews. The word ghetto, which is used by sociologists and other scholars to describe segregated residential areas, originally was used to describe the Jewish section of European cities. It is believed that the word had its origin in Venice, which in the late Middle Ages had set apart a portion of the city as the Jewish quarter.[9] This ghettoization of Jews in Europe had been partly voluntary (for religious and cultural reasons), partly protective (because of periodic outbreaks of hostility to Jews), but mainly for legal reasons. As the Jewish communities had grown and the boundaries had remained unchanged, the European ghettos cramped more and more people into a small space. Ghettoization also prevented the Jews' assimilation into the general culture of the surrounding communities, and in fact, large numbers of Jews in Poland and Russia did not speak the languages of these countries but instead spoke Yiddish.

With this background, Jewish immigrants came to the United States already prepared for ghetto life. They settled primarily in the large urban areas, with New York City serving as the home of more than half of the new Jewish immigrants.[10] Though there had been earlier waves of Jewish settlers from Spain and Portugal (via Brazil) and from Germany, after 1881 the largest groups came from Russia (including Poland) as refugees from the periodic pogroms and other persecutions. The already existing Jewish community helped the poverty-stricken refugees survive, but it also helped cut them off from contact with other ethnic groups. Orthodox Jews—and most of the immigrants were Orthodox—were not supposed to ride to the synagogue on the sabbath, and this meant that the devoted Jew could not move far from the synagogue. Successful second- and third-generation descendents of the immigrants who wanted to move out into more comfortable neighborhoods, yet remain Jewish, were forced to move the synagogue with them or change their religion to suit the realities of American life. Both of these things took place, with Conservative and Reform Judaism developing, but the nature of the European experience in the ghetto and the outside pressures of the non-Jewish community made the assimilation of Jewish minorities slower than some of the other groups.[11] They also suffered greater discrimination in jobs, housing, public accomodation than their Christian countrymen who were often contemporary immigrants. College fraternities and sororities, for example, long excluded Jews because they were non-Christian, even in non-sectarian state universities. Many colleges and universities put a quota on entrance for non-Christians.

The Growth of Racism and the Control of Immigration

The wave of Jewish immigrants was just part of a flood of people seeking new opportunities in the United States. In the decade between 1900 and 1910 immigration reached a peak as more than eight million people arrived in the United States. Inevitably the great waves of immigrants created hostility to the open-immigration policy and there was a growing "racism" toward the newer immigrants. As the Indians were the only indigenous Americans, it became necessary to rationalize the hostility on grounds other than simple immigrant status. To this end science, or rather pseudoscience, contributed a new justification. Sociology, which was only beginning to emerge as an independent discipline, made generalizations about the immigrant which have proved shocking to the sociologist of today. Nevertheless, through analyzing criminality, intemperance, poverty, and disease, these early sociologists found that the immigrant was associated with all social problems. This meant that either society was at fault or the newcomer, and it proved much too tempting to blame the problems on the immigrant himself. Sociologists adopted the dictum that social characteristics were dependent upon racial differences and a succession of books were published demonstrating that the flaws in the biological constitution of the newer immigrants were responsible for every evil that beset America— from pauperism, to depression, to homosexuality. Historians, novelists, and politicians joined this movement and a body of literature grew up expounding the innate biological superiority of Northern Europeans with the corollary argument that all other peoples were of physically and/or mentally inferior stock.[12] Joining with the emerging social scientist in the racist cause were labor union leaders who saw the new immigrant as a means for employers to undercut wages and undermine the craftsmen who then dominated organized labor.

The first group actually to be restricted were the Chinese, with passage of the Exclusion Act in 1882, which many of its supporters regarded as only temporary. The legislation was passed in response to the virulent anti-Chinese feelings of Californians, who were convinced that the Chinese "coolies" were suppressing wages. Local discriminatory legislation had been passed earlier and the Chinese residents had been subjected to numerous incidents of mob violence. Rather than a temporary act, however, the Chinese Exclusion Act proved a harbinger of things to come. In 1894 the Immigration Restriction League was formed in Boston to limit the number of admissions and to select from among the potential applicants only the superior stocks related to the "American Aryans." Various prohibited categories were adopted. In 1882 Congress had also barred idiots, criminals, and others likely to become public charges. In 1891 this had been extended to take in believers in anarchism and in polygamy (aimed at the Mormons), as well as contract laborers. Adding to the anti-immigrant pressure was the fear of radicalism by the business community, a fear sparked by the Haymarket Riot in 1886 when five of the six anarchists accused of the bombing that killed several policemen proved to be immigrants. World War I emphasized the xenophobic tendencies in America, and when "100 percent Americanism" was the order of the day it was dangerous to champion the cause of the foreign-born. In 1917, over the veto of President Woodrow Wilson, the literacy test was enacted into law, requiring every newcomer to the United States to demonstrate his ability to read. It was assumed by its sponsors that this would bar the southern and eastern Europeans without excluding those from the northern and western parts of the continent where the facilities for elementary education had become much more common by 1917. Such a differentiation was advocated because it conformed to the racist assumptions of the sponsors, but it was also politically strategic because it sought the support of those foreign-born groups that were not adversely affected.

Since the Chinese remained the only national group which was totally excluded by name, many Christian missionaries sought to remove the exclusion provisions of the immigration legislation because it proved a handicap to them in their missionary efforts. Earlier it had been proposed to admit a percentage of immigrants equal to the natives already resident in the United States as an alternative to use of the literacy test, and this system in the mind of several missionary leaders had the advantage of not being aimed at Orientals in particular.

In 1921 Congress adopted a scheme providing for limiting the newcomers to 3 percent of the number from their nation who were living in the United States in 1910. But under this formula Asiatics still received harsh treatment, and this heightened rather than eased antagonisms in the Orient. In 1924 a further restriction was imposed because the quotas were based upon the proportion of residents present in the population in 1890—which was before the large-scale Polish, Russian, Italian, and Jewish immigration occurred. This act also completely excluded Japanese immigrants.

With the 1924 act, the period of mass migration into the United States basically ended and even the anti-Jewish pogroms of Adolf Hitler did not change the system. Millions of Jews were killed who might have lived had the United States been willing to amend its immigration policy to accept refugees.

In spite of pressure, however, it was not until 1952 that the United States modified the immigration law to allow refugees as well as a few Asians to enter the country legally; most of the Asians who became citizens under this provision had been residents of the United States for much of their life. More important was the refugee provision which allowed Hungarians, Cubans, and others caught up in the turmoil of the post-World War II period to be admitted. In 1965, there was a further modification so that unfilled quotas based on the percentage of nationals in the population in 1890 could be used by "preference" immigrants whose national quotas had been exhausted. Preference immigrants were those who would be reunited with their families or who had skills and talents needed in the country. It was this provision which led the so-called "undeveloped" countries to complain of a brain drain since so many physicians, scientists, and other such professionals were allowed to become citizens of the United States rather than return to their homeland after completing schooling. In 1968 there was a further revision, with a yearly limit of 170,000 set for immigrants from countries outside the Western Hemisphere with a 20,000 maximum from any one country, and a total of 120,000 immigrants from the Western Hemisphere to be admitted on a first-come-first-served basis.

The Health of the Immigrants

Most of the immigrants arrived in America in an exhausted state, worn out by lack of rest, by poor food, by the cramped quarters on ships, and unaccustomed to new conditions. In the early part of the 19th century, sea travel itself was exhausting. The journey from Liverpool to New York averaged about 40 days, although favorable winds might lower it somewhat and unfavorable ones might raise it to two or three months. Wrecks were frequent and disastrous. In one year in the 1830s 17 vessels foundered on the run from Liverpool to Quebec alone. Fire was an ever-present danger, and so was disease. Great numbers of immigrants came steerage class and vessels before the Civil War were pitifully small, some three hundred tons, crammed with anywhere from four hundred to a thousand passengers. Though there were cabins for the well-to-do, most travelers lived below decks in the hold which was about seventy-five feet long, twenty-five feet wide, and only about six feet high. Each family received a daily ration of water to which they added larger and larger doses of vinegar to conceal the odor. In steerage the passengers furnished their own provisions, and if they ran out they either went hungry or had to buy from the ship's captain at prices they could ill afford. It was not until mid-century that the United States government would specify the supplies which had to be taken on for each passenger.[13]

The only ventilation below the deck was through the hatches, which were battened down in rough weather. When the air was not stifling hot, it was bitter cold in the absence of fire. Rats were at home in the dirt and disorder. The result was cholera, dysentery, yellow fever, smallpox, measles, and a sort of generic "ship fever" that might be anything. The normal mortality on crossing was about 10 percent, although some years it was closer to 20 percent. Some changes for the better came in mid-century. The introduction of steam in the 1840s and the appearance of the Cunard Line and its imitators took over the upper-class passenger business and left the immigrant trade to the sailing ships, which were consequently forced to improve accomodations. After 1870 the new emphasis on merchant fleets led France, Germany, England, and Italy to build larger ships and to give subsidies to the operators of lines bearing their flags. Under these circumstances the price of steerage passage on a steamship fell to as little as twelve dollars and included food. By 1900 the traveler could count on a crossing of little more than a week in vessels of ten to twenty thousand tons. It was still not an easy trip since the ships were overcrowded, there was lack of privacy, and the food was poor, but much larger proportions survived the voyage. Still, it is no wonder that so many were so exhausted that they stayed at the port of embarkation without going on into the interior. Those who did move on used the railroads and often remained at the junction points on the route—e.g., Buffalo, Cleveland, Pittsburgh, Chicago, St. Louis, and Milwaukee—even though they had originally intended to go elsewhere.

Increasingly, in fact, the immigrant came to settle in the cities, and rural small town America saw proportionately fewer of the new masses of people that came in the last part of the 19th and first part of the 20th century. This occurred in spite of the fact that great numbers of immigrants had originally left with the intention of farming and tilling the soil. In fact unless they had money and resources, or organized expeditions (as the Mormons did), few of them managed to escape from the cities. Most of them, even though of peasant origin and knowing only how to farm, became trapped in the city, able only to sell their strength since they had little of the skills needed for other jobs. It was the immigrant who built the canals, and the railroads, and the early highways which in the days before big earth-moving equipment was available required masses of men. The factories and mines also offered employment opportunities, and some immigrants became machine operators. Many also opened businesses to serve their fellow immigrants as storekeepers, butchers, bakers, and so forth.

Trapped in the city, however, life was still hard and death rates were high. New York City and the other major Atlantic ports, where the immigrant concentration was greatest, crowded newcomers into tenements. In the interior of the country smaller units were more the norm, but it was not unusual to stuff six families into places built for one. This overcrowding helped to spread disease; tuberculosis rates were particularly high among the foreign-born population. The immigrants were also pushed into the least desirable places to live. In Chicago it was over against the slaughterhouses, in Boston they were hemmed in by the docks and markets of the North End, and in other towns they located near the railroad switching yard. One of the great problems in tenements was that of sanitation. Many of the early buildings had been built without privies at all. From the mid-century onward most tenements were built with privies or water closets (which washed away the sewage) that were located outside in the backyards and alleys. For those people who lived on the sixth floor, this arrangement was inconvenient to say the least. Later on, as the modern flush toilet was developed, the newer tenements were built with inside toilets, usually two on each floor. These were, however, open to all comers, but charged to the care of none and left to the neglect of all. In the winter the pipes overflowed, and weeks might go by before matters were set right. Some of the tenements thereafter retained the odor of human excrement through the rest of their history.

Filth was inescapable. Open drains were common, and even in a city as large as Chicago, it was not until well into the 20th century that some of the sewers were covered, so that until that time fly-borne diseases were quite prevalent. As an adequate water supply was difficult to obtain, it was often necessary to carry tubs and jugs from taps in the alley. Water was connected to toilets first, and in many cases water for drinking and bathing still had to be carried from a public faucet outside. Illness was rampant, drunkenness was common, and behavioral disorders and neuroses—all classed as "insanity" in that day—were ever-present. America, however, was slow to deal with the problems. The New York State Senate in 1858 appointed a committee to look into the need for municipal health measures. It attributed the high rate of mortality in New York City at that time to the

> overcrowded condition of tenement houses, the want of practical knowledge of the proper mode of constructing such houses, deficiency of light, imperfect ventilation, impurities in domestic economy, unwholesome food and beverages, insufficient sewage [i.e. sewers], want of cleanliness in the streets and at the wharves and piers, to a general disregard of sanitary precautions, and finally, to the imperfect execution of existing ordinances and the total absence of a regularly organized sanitary police.[14]

Finally, in 1866, the Metropolitan Board of Health was established, and soon after this New York City was given its own department. Much of the early activity of the Board was motivated by the concept that disease was caused by dirt, and investigators concentrated on reporting defective plumbing or ventilation, and tried to control contagious disease through environmental sanitation.

Immigrants, and slum dwellers in particular, were hard hit by the various epidemics which hit the United States in the 19th century. Cholera epidemics hit in 1832, 1848 to 1849, 1866, and 1873. Yellow fever was more or less endemic during much of the 19th century, as was smallpox. Diphtheria and scarlet fever were major causes of death among children, and during the 40-year period of 1840 to 1880, scarlet fever was particularly virulent.

Actual control of the contagious diseases was dependent upon the development of the germ theory by Louis Pasteur and others during the last part of the 19th century. The new science of bacteriology reached the United States in the 1880s and gradually more effective preventive measures were taken against epidemics.

The epidemics, as well as illness in general, were more likely to hit the immigrant than the more affluent Americans primarily because of the nature of the living conditions. However, medical care of the poor was also inferior to that given to the more well-to-do people. Hospitals were primarily charitable institutions, as we have indicated; they were not particularly clean, and through most of the 19th century they lacked any kind of trained nursing care. As we stated in Chapter 1, well-to-do people were cared for by servants or by physicians themselves—at home where there was less chance of the spread of infection.[15]

Communities did little to care for the health needs of the poor. In 1859 the New York Infirmary for Women and Children appointed a "sanitary visitor" to give simple practical instruction to "poor mothers on the management of infants, and the preservation of the health of families," but this effort was soon submerged in the Civil War. During the Panic (or depression) of 1873, the New York Diet Kitchen set up food stations to feed the poor, and as conditions improved the food station became a milk station for babies. The most effective effort in this direction, however, was by the private philanthropist, Nathan Strauss, who in 1893 established a system of milk stations which by 1902 were distributing 250,000 bottles monthly. The settlement house movement was also important in bettering conditions, serving in a sense as the modern community clinic. A settlement house differed from other social agencies in that it was concerned about the neighborhood as a whole. It sought to develop relationships among the community groups of different cultural, religious, and social characteristics, and to help people act together to improve their living conditions and environment. The two most famous settlements—both of which were opened at the end of the 19th century—were Hull House in Chicago, started by Jane Addams and Ellen Gates Starr, and the Henry Street Settlement in New York, started by two nurses, Lillian Wald and Mary Brewster.[16] Both settlements emphasized health care and education, and did much to develop the professions of social work and public health nursing. Though the settlement house movement, and particularly Hull House and the Henry Street Settlement, are now looked upon with universal favor and even reverence, in their own day they were considered to be quite radical. They helped to develop autonomous neighborhood organizations, and the women involved saw the poverty of the immigrants as something which could be corrected. Both Lillian Wald and Jane Addams were politically oriented and urged protective labor legislation, child welfare laws, compensation for working men when injured, and various other forms of government intervention to deal with the problems of the poor, all of which were regarded as alien and radical ideas by the more affluent segment of society.

Half a century has passed since the end of the large-scale European migration to this country, and new minority groups have emerged. Some of the problems faced by these new groups are similar to those encountered by the European immigrants, although there are some essential differences between them and those faced by the Negroes, the Mexican-Americans, and the Puerto Ricans who are the major minority groups on the current scene. However, some knowledge of past patterns and events helps to put both the similarities and the differences in context.

Notes

1. Louis Wirth, "The Problem of Minority Groups," *The Science of Man in the World Crisis,* edited by Ralph Linton (New York: Columbia University Press, 1945), pp. 345-372.
2. Frank Julian Warne, *The Tide of Immigration* (New York: D. Appleton and Co., 1916), p. 205.
3. A. M. Carr-Saunders, *World Population* (Oxford: Clarendon Press, 1936), p. 49.
4. Maldwyn Allen Jones, *American Immigration* (Chicago: University of Chicago Press, 1960), pp. 22-27.
5. *Ibid.,* p. 49.
6. Lillian Wald, *The House on Henry Street* (New York: Henry Holt and Co., 1915), pp. 1-25; Ernest W. Burgess, "Urban Areas," *Chicago: An Experiment in Social Science Research,* edited by T. V. Smith and Leonard White (Chicago: University of Chicago Press, 1929), pp. 113-138.
7. Colin Greer, "Public Schools: The Myth of the Melting Pot," *Saturday Review* (November 15, 1969), pp. 84-86, 102-103.
8. Jones, *op. cit.,* p. 43.
9. Louis Wirth, *The Ghetto* (Chicago: University of Chicago Press, 1928), p. 2.
10. *Ibid.,* pp. 150-151.
11. Milton Gordon, *Assimilation in American Life: The Role of Race, Religion, and National Origin* (New York: Oxford University Press, 1964), p. 123 *passim.*
12. Thomas F. Gossett, *Race: The History of an Idea in America* (Dallas: Southern Methodist University Press, 1963), pp. 287-309.

13. Oscar Handlin, *The Uprooted* (Boston: Atlantic-Little, Brown, 1952), pp. 37-62.
14. George Rosen, *A History of Public Health* (New York: MD Publications, 1958), p. 244.
15. Vern and Bonnie Bullough, *Emergence of Modern Nursing*, 2nd edition (New York: Macmillan, 1969), pp. 120-148.
16. Wald, *op. cit.*, and Jane Addams, *Twenty Years at Hull House* (New York: Macmillan, 1912).

3

Black Americans

The modern business and industrial complex has, since its beginnings in the 18th century, depended upon a supply of cheap labor to carry out the more burdensome and lower-paying tasks. Traditionally, workers to perform these jobs have been recruited from the farm and the village. When rural areas were not able to meet the demands for workers countries such as England turned to parts of their Empire, particularly to Ireland, but in recent years West Indians, Pakistani, and Indians have come to England in great numbers. Other countries such as Germany and Switzerland have since World War II recruited large numbers of Italians, Greeks, Yugoslavs, and people from other nations where industrialization has not been so advanced. Most of these workers sign to work for a stipulated length of time and leave their families behind. In a sense they are today's counterpart to the sojourners and other temporary immigrants to the United States in the past.

In the United States industrial workers have traditionally come from the small towns and the farm or from among the recent immigrants. Since World War I and the passage of the laws restricting immigration, the movement from the farm to the city has been speeded up, both because of the demands for workers and because of the mechanization of the farm, which has tended to make the lot of the small farmer more and more difficult. Not all sections of the United States have undergone industrialization at the same pace, and in general the greatest industrialization has taken place along the coastal areas and around the Great Lakes. This has meant that migration within the United States, at least in the 20th century, has not only been from the farm to the city but also from the South, one of the poorer and least industrialized sections of the country, to the North and West, and from the farm belt in the interior of the country to coastal and Great Lakes centers of industry.

In general those residents of the rural areas most likely to move to the city were either the young, the dissatisfied, or those who lacked property and investment. Inevitably many of them went through periods of readjustment which were as severe as those faced by immigrants from other countries. The so-called "Oakies" and "Arkies" who migrated to California during the '20s and '30s were met with hostility and exploitation. Their culture seemed to the Californians at the time to be almost an alien one.[1] Facing even greater prejudice in their migration northward were the Negroes who were not only less educated than the "Oakies" but also had the difficulty of skin color and the burden of past slavery to overcome. Replacing the "Oakies" of the '30s as the most poverty-stricken section of white America, are the residents of Appalachia, many of whom have moved to the city seeking employment as the coal fields and farms of Appalachia began to fail.

Another source of cheap labor, both in the city and in the country, are the Spanish-speaking migrants from Puerto Rico, who are American citizens, and those from Mexico, who cross the border both legally and illegally to find work. There are also large numbers of indigenous Spanish-speaking peoples in the Southwest whose territory had been annexed to the United States in the 19th century, some of whom still lack real facility in English. Still another indigenous group with real minority status are the native Americans, the Indians, many of whom live in poverty on reservations or in the slums of the city. Other visible minorities such as the Oriental Americans also face problems but economically both the Japanese and Chinese Americans are better off than the Negroes, the Spanish-speaking Americans, or the Indians. The reasons for the difficulties faced by the various groups is in part explained by an examination of the way in which they have arrived at their present position. The remainder of this chapter will be devoted to discussing the Negroes.

The Negroes

Blacks had come to America early, perhaps with Columbus, although there is some scholarly dispute as to whether Pedro Alonzo Nino, the navigator of the Niña was a Negro or not. It is known for certain that several members of the French and Spanish exploring parties were Negroes, and Jean Baptiste Point Du Sable, the founder of Chicago, for example, was a Negro.[2] The overwhelming majority of Africans who came to this country, however, were different from other immigrants in that they came unwillingly on slave ships. Slavery was big business in American colonial history and many a New England fortune was built upon the transportation of slaves from the West Indies, where they had been brought by the British. During the 17th century Dutch, French, Portuguese, and English companies were the mainstay of the slave trade from Africa, but by the 18th century the English had achieved dominance.

Slaves were captured or bought from Arab tradesmen in West Africa—primarily from the Gold Coast (modern Ghana) or the Congo. They were then chained together and packed into ships for the passage across the Atlantic, and although the mortality rate for European immigrants was high, that of black slaves was much higher. In fact, everything that the willing European immigrant had faced was compounded for the Negro who faced greater overcrowding, less adequate food, and a general feeling of hopelessness. Probably no more than half of the slaves who were loaded on the ships in Africa actually reached their destination, at least in any condition which would enable them to become effective workers. Large numbers died of disease, committed suicide, or were permanently disabled either by the ravages of disease or from the injuries they received. Profits were so great, however, that traders made little effort to reform their brutal practices but rather simply stuffed more people into their ships to compensate for their expected losses.

It was the development of the sugar crop in the Caribbean islands which had first made the American slave trade so profitable and it was the West Indies which served as the destination of the early slave ships. Here slaves were "seasoned" or taught their new work roles under the whips of overseers. It was from the West Indies that the slaves were transported to the American colonies, a trade which rapidly increased after 1792 with the invention of the cotton gin. Cotton became an important money crop in the South at the very time that sugar was becoming less important in the West Indies.

To America's credit there were always powerful critics of the slave trade, and they managed to abolish the practice in the United States as of January 1, 1808. Great Britain abolished it first in 1806 but in stronger terms in 1811. Since the British controlled the seas as well as the west coast of Africa, their effort to abolish the trade proved particularly effective and by the middle of the 19th century, it had been nearly eliminated. The elimination of the slave trade removed one abuse, but it did not necessarily improve the lot of the slave who now had to work harder. Moreover, some of the areas of the United States took to encouraging the breeding of slaves, selling the surplus to other areas. The abolition of the slave trade also did not end the practice of hiring contract laborers whom the British recruited in India, China, and elsewhere and transported to various ports. Contract laborers from China, for example, built the western portion of the transcontinental railroad across the United States. Though nominally under contract, in fact many of the indentured laborers were recruited by unscrupulous means, and all too often their contracts for return to their homeland were not honored.

It was the British, nonetheless, who led the effort to eliminate actual slavery. In 1833 slavery was officially abolished in British possessions, although the act was only to take place after slaves had been trained to take jobs in society. In the British West Indies, for example, it was not until 1838 that all slaves were free. Gradually other European states followed the British example, with France emancipating its slaves in 1848, Portugal in 1858, and Holland in 1863, although in most cases freedom was given only gradually. Mexico abolished slavery in 1829 and Brazil in 1871, but the full effect was not felt in Brazil until 1888. Slavery continued to exist in the Spanish possessions of Cuba and Puerto

Rico in the Caribbean and in the Philippines in the Pacific until these colonies were taken over or given their independence by the United States as a result of the Spanish American War.

In the United States the struggle for emancipation was long and bitter, and extremely divisive, mainly because slavery was not particularly profitable in New England, the Middle Atlantic States, or the developing West, and thus it came to be a phenomenon largely concentrated in the South. Moreover, the fact that emancipation occurred only in conjunction with the Civil War undoubtedly made the life of the Negro freedman much more difficult than it might have been if the owners had been given compensation as they had in the British colonies. All this left its trauma on the American Negro.

Impact of Slavery

Scholars are not in full agreement about the impact of slavery on the culture of the American Negro, although the disagreement is probably more apparent than real. Franklin Frazier, a pioneer Negro sociologist, held that the trauma of the terrifying trip across the Atlantic, the brutal breaking-in experience in the West Indies or under the American plantation overseers, plus the humiliating experience of slavery itself, virtually destroyed the African cultural heritage. The surviving remnants were further weakened by the fact that slaves were forced to use English to communicate with each other because their tribal origins and languages varied so much, and individuals from the same tribe were usually separated from each other in order to cut down the dangers of insurrection.[3] Slavery also destroyed the African family system since slaves were forbidden to marry. While free unions between men and women were undoubtedly formed, they could be violated by the owners of the slave who could seize a woman for his own sexual pleasure or break up a potential family by selling off some of its members. Inevitably the collective personality shaped by these experiences had little resemblance to the proud and independent African tribesmen who had been the slave's ancestor.[4]

Anthropologists, led by Melville Herskovits, held that even though the experiences recounted by Frazier were true, the

Negroes still managed to retain some of their past tradition. Herskovits studied African culture traits and compared them with Negro culture traits in the New World, and found similarities in language, religion, music, and numerous other aspects of culture. Though the slaves learned English, they used African patterns in speech and intonation, and managed to keep alive folks tales and magical practices which they brought with them from Africa. Such carryovers, however, were more evident in the West Indies and in Latin America than in the large urban ghettoes of the American North.[5]

Increasingly, as studies on Africa and the Negro have progressed, there has emerged a kind of concensus. Even though the slave was brutally removed from his past and thrust unwillingly into a radically different life pattern, and denied opportunities to form associations to preserve fond memories, he still undoubtedly viewed his experience from the point of view of his past, and his culture was vibrant enough and engrained enough to allow him to do so. In fact, the rich cultural heritage of the American Negro, however brutalized he might have been, has enriched all of American culture.

The End of Slavery

Emancipation of the slaves, however, did not end the problems of the Negro. Although slavery was abolished in the aftermath of the Civil War, few of the Negroes were educated, and many of them had picked up "survival traits" in slavery which made adjustment in a nonslave society difficult. Moreover, the bulk of the white South was accustomed to Negroes as slaves, and they were determined to assert their dominance over the blacks who in many parts of the South outnumbered the whites. When Negroes, with the encouragement of the federal government and the presence of Union troops, assumed positions of authority, the South countered by establishing secret movements designed to keep the Negro down, by terror if necessary. The Knights of the White Camelia and Ku-Klux Klan were the most powerful of the secret orders and armed with guns, swords, and other weapons the members patrolled some parts of the South day and night. Scattered Union troops proved wholly ineffectual in coping with the problem, and few Negroes were able to face up to the threats. Many either left the South or resigned themselves to trying to seek advancement through other ways. Those Negroes who did go North found that they were greeted with hostility and suspicion because most of the northerners, while antislavery, were also anti-Negro.

Though the dedicated abolitionists made attempts to ensure Negro rights in the South, they were comparatively few in number. Even though the southerners had lost the war, they were determined to rule themselves, and they believed in their minds and hearts that the Negroes were not qualified to rule. As the restraints imposed upon the southerners by the federal government and the presence of occupying troops were relaxed or removed, and the stringent postwar legislation repealed, the Reconstruction of the South gradually fell into the hands of the southerners, and while there were occasionally bloody racial clashes, the white southerner soon emerged dominant. In the aftermath of the disputed presidential election of 1876 between Rutherford B. Hayes and Samuel J. Tilden, an agreement was made by the Republicans to withdraw all federal troops in return for southern electoral support of Hayes. By this time the North had grown weary of the crusade for Negro rights, and while there were still some old antislavery leaders, most of the leaders of the younger generation had little zeal for the Negro and cared more about the industrial and business interests in the North and South. With the return of the old leaders in the South, most of whom identified with the Democratic party, ways were soon found to disenfranchise Negroes or to nullify their political strength in spite of the Fifteenth Amendment to the Constitution. As soon as the political power of the Negroes and their allies declined the South turned to erecting the barrier of segregation to replace the old barrier of slavery. This so-called "Jim Crow" legislation separated blacks and whites on trains, in depots, on wharves, in barber shops, restaurants, theaters, schools, and in almost every aspect of life. This was not done without opposition, but the southern officials either executed or expelled those Negroes who opposed the imposition of segregation. In the first two years of the 20th century there were some 214 lynchings of Negroes in the South, and with the law, the courts, and the execution of justice in the hands of whites, Negroes, even though technically no longer slaves, had to struggle just to survive, and could only make feeble gropings in the direction of progress.[6]

Trends Within the Negro Community

It was in this situation that Booker T. Washington rose to prominence. Washington, who had become head of the Tuskegee Institute in 1881, believed that southern whites in particular had to be convinced that the education of the Negro was in the true interest of the South. In a rather fatherly fashion he counseled Negroes to respect the law, cooperate with the white authorities in maintaining peace, and to train themselves to become farmers, mechanics, and domestic servants until they had improved themselves sufficiently to be ready for better things. Washington taught habits of thrift, patience, perserverance, the cultivation of good manners, and in the process won the support of many southern whites as well as northerners who saw his plan as a formula for peace in the South. Though Washington believed in the ultimate attainment of acceptance and integration, many of his white supporters, skeptical of the capacity of the Negro to become completely assimilated, viewed his scheme as leading the Negro to his proper place in American life, a position which they felt should be inferior to that of the whites. Others of his white supporters were so happy with his gradualism that they never bothered about his ultimate goals.

One of the leading opponents of the Washington philosophy was W. E. B. DuBois, a Harvard-educated, northern-born Negro, who went South to teach and to do research on the Negroes. DuBois believed that it was impossible for Negroes, no matter what their level in society, to defend themselves without the vote. He also held that Washington's advice to the Negroes to stay in rural areas did not face up to the reality of the ongoing industrialization and urbanization in America. In 1905 a group of Negro men under the leadership of DuBois, determined to secure full citizenship, met in conference at Niagara Falls, Canada. They wrote a platform which demanded freedom of speech and criticism, suffrage, abolition of all distinctions based on race, recognition of basic principles of human brotherhood, and respect for the workingman. The group called itself the Niagara Movement and planned for periodic meetings. Following a race riot in Springfield, Illinois, in August 1908, they joined with various old surviving abolition movements, and other groups interested in bettering the lot of the Negro, to hold a conference on Lincoln's birthday in 1909. Out of this came the National Association for the Advancement of Colored People (NAACP), most of whose first officers were white. The organization of the NAACP was followed in 1911 by the National Urban League. The NAACP and to a lesser extent the Urban League led the battle for more effective integration of the American Negro.

Integration, however, was a slow and difficult process, and not all Negroes were agreed upon the aims of the NAACP. In fact, the NAACP failed for the most part to touch the imagination of the masses. Negroes on the lower social and economic level, if they knew of it or similar organizations, were inclined to regard them as agencies of upper-class Negroes or of liberal whites who were not particularly aware of the economic necessities of remaining alive. Much more popular for a time was the Universal Negro Improvement Association founded by Marcus Garvey in 1914. Garvey exalted everthing black, and insisted that black stood for strength and beauty, not inferiority. He asserted that Africans had a noble past of which Negroes should be proud. He also held that the only hope for Negroes was to flee America and to return to Africa where they could build a country of their own. His appeal struck a responsive chord and his followers numbered in the millions for a time in the 1920s. Garvey's movement collapsed not because of Negro disillusionment with what he advocated, but because of his own personal failures. He was accused of using the mails to defraud in raising money to run his steamship line to take Negroes to Africa, and in 1925 he was sent to jail under a five-year sentence. When he was pardoned, he returned to his native Jamaica, and his movement was dead.

The history of the American Negro in the 20th century in part has been a conflict between the dualism expressed by DuBois and Garvey. One segment has pushed for integration, while the other has emphasized black power and ties with Africa. The Washington philosophy has little current following and the most ignored of Washington's program has been his advice to stay on the farm, as is evident from the census figures. In 1910, 73 percent of the Negro population were rural, and overwhelmingly southern. By 1960, 73 percent were urban, and more Negroes lived outside the South than in it.[7] Although in one sense the Negroes are among the oldest immigrants, the change from the rural south to the urbanized industrialized north has been so dramatic that in effect they have gone through a second immigration.

It was in the period following the outbreak of World War I that large-scale Negro migration into the northern industrial cities really began to mushroom, a movement that is still underway. In the process Negroes have come to have a politically potent voice in the North, and as they have become a political force, gained access to better education, and to some of the better-paying jobs. Negro militancy has increased. Nondiscriminatory provisions were required of defense industries in World War II, and this was followed by the passage of Fair Employment Practice Acts in many states, and finally by the United States Government itself. The NAACP and some of the other civil rights and civil liberties groups had turned to the courts to redress some of the most outrageous forms of discrimination against Negroes and in the period from World War II to today whole series of laws have been declared unconstitutional—including restrictive convenants in housing, segregated interstate transportation, and separate but equal schools. Declaring a law unconstitutional and achieving equality were, however, often different things and beginning in the 1950s a whole series of civil rights agitations led to actual enforcement of some of the constitutional provisions giving equality. Martin Luther King, Jr., in 1956 rose to fame and leadership through his role in the Montgomery, Alabama, bus boycott. Sit-in demonstrations at lunch counters led to the integration of many southern restaurants, and Congress itself through various Civil Rights Acts attempted to remove the remaining barriers against discrimination. The result has been a period of turmoil and increasing militancy on behalf of the Negroes as they realized that much of the suffering they had endured in the past was no longer necessary: Inevitably there have been riots as ghettoes rebelled at the continuing forms of discrimination, and these riots originally confined to Negro areas have spread to areas of other minority groups, particularly the Spanish-speaking Americans.

Inequalities in Health and Health Care

One of the areas in which the past history of discrimination, repression, and suspicion has most effectively left its mark upon the Negro of today, is in the area of health care. Data on life expectancy which have been available since 1900 indicate that there has been a persistent gap between the expected length of life of the white and the nonwhite population (94 percent of those so classified are Negro). Table 1 shows these life expectancies by decade. Although the gap has narrowed as the health of the total population has improved, there are still significant differences

TABLE 1. Life expectancy at birth for white and nonwhite population[8]

Year	White	Nonwhite
1900	47.6	33.0
1910	50.3	35.6
1920	54.9	45.3
1930	61.4	48.1
1940	64.2	53.1
1950	69.1	60.8
1960	70.6	63.6
1967	71.3	64.6

From United States Department of Health, Education, and Welfare, Vital Statistics of the United States, 1967, Vol., II *(Washington, D.C.: U.S. Government Printing Office, 1968), Table 5-6.*

between the two groups. It is not only segregation and discrimination which have produced these differences in health but also poverty, lack of education, and the negative psychological responses that follow from these difficulties. If it were necessary to rank these variables, poverty would undoubtedly come first, but in a sense, this is misleading because poverty is inextricably intertwined with all forms of discrimination, each difficulty reinforcing the other. Nevertheless, when one uses the index of poverty developed by the Social Security Administration, 35 percent of the nation's nonwhite families fall below the poverty line, and there are almost an equal number who live in what is called "near" poverty. On the other hand, only 10 percent of the white population can be classified as falling below the poverty line, and about the same percentage belong in the "near" poverty group.[9] Since the aged make up a large proportion of the poor white group, poverty among young families is more of a minority group phenomenon. This is important in assessing health care because neglect of the current health needs of the nonwhite children can have long-term consequences for their health even if as adults they are fortunate enough to escape the cycle of poverty.

Part of the explanation for the poverty of the nonwhite population is found in the lower educational level of the Negroes, but the problem is really more complex than it looks on the surface. Job discrimination has lessened since the passage of state and federal legislation outlawing such practices, but it still is an important factor in holding back the Negro worker. Moreover, the nature of industry in the United States has changed during the last two or three decades so that there is less of a demand for the unskilled worker than in the past. As industry has become more and more mechanized, or as the cybernetic revolution has gathered momentum, jobs for unskilled workers have become more and more difficult to obtain.

Even with an education, however, black workers still face tremendous disadvantages. Many of the craft unions, traditionally the province of the highest-skilled and highest-paid workers, have until recently denied admission of visible minority groups into their membership. Moreover, the segregated educational system gives black students an education that is of lower quality than that received by white counterparts who spent the same number of years in school. There are also more subtle kinds of discrimination: the black worker may have been hired at the entry level but overlooked for advancement. The result has been a gap between the income of the white and black workers. The gap is narrowest between those Negroes and whites who have less than an eighth grade education or a college or graduate degree. It is greatest between those who have attended or graduated from high school or who have attended a junior college.[10] Only a comparatively few Negroes have graduated from college, and as jobs become difficult to find, the differential rate of unemployment increases. In 1960, for example, the unemployment rate for white workers was 4.7 percent while 8.7 percent of the black workers were unemployed.[11] At other times during the past decade the rate of unemployment has been almost two-and-a-half times higher than whites, and in the large urban ghetto of Watts in Los Angeles it has gone to three times as high. Unemployment in the concentrated ghetto areas is particularly serious during periods of recession because many of the workers are unskilled.[12] Inevitably there are hundreds of young men in their 20s who, though long finished with their schooling, have never held a job, or have held only a temporary training job under the Office of Economic Opportunities programs. Cut off from highly skilled jobs by lack of education and by discrimination, Negroes are often denied the opportunity to work at all because the need for unskilled workmen is dwindling. In fact, it is the changing nature of the employment which most differentiates the current minority populations from the earlier European immigrants. Though the newly arrived European also suffered from poverty, discrimination, and even segregation, they were able to find employment. Then with hard work, and a certain amount of luck, they or their children were able to move up the occupational ladder. Now the bottom rung of the ladder is being cut off.

Obviously unemployed people or people whose incomes are below or near the poverty line cannot buy medical care on the open market. Since our health care delivery system is based on the ability of an individual to pay for the care he gets, the poor are in effect cut off from much of the benefit of modern medical development, and this at a time when health care has become crucially important to survival. Before the 20th century, medical intervention was not necessarily a significant factor in determining life expectancy; diet, sanitation, and other aspects of the environment were far more important in explaining the differential life expectancies between the rich and the poor. Today, however, medical care itself is a major factor in determining life expectancy, and this means that regardless of whether a person is able to buy, good medical care becomes of overriding concern. Most of the advanced European countries, realizing that health care itself had become such an important factor in life expectancy, made the decision to make it available, through various kinds of schemes, to all residents regardless of their socioeconomic status. In the United States, the richest country in the world with the best educated medical profession, health care has remained essentially a fee-for-service commodity, which means that those who do not have the fee cannot get the essential life-saving service.

Problems of Voluntary Health Care

This is not to say that some positive steps have not been taken. Voluntary prepaid health insurance has softened the impact of the system for most Americans. In 1963, 88 percent of the families whose income was over $7,000 carried some form of hospital and surgical insurance, and almost as great a percentage, some 79 percent, of those whose incomes were between $4,000 and $7,000 had some form of coverage. Only 52 percent of the families with incomes between $2,000 and $4,000 were insured, and 34 percent of those with family incomes below $2,000 were covered.[13] Obviously the type of coverage varied, and in actuality comparatively few had policies which would pay for all of their medical costs. In spite of these qualifications, however, the average white was better off than the black, simply because the majority of nonwhite families had no hospital insurance at all or had totally inadequate coverage. This means that they were outside of the voluntary health care delivery system.

Americans, perhaps uncomfortably conscious of the fact that not all people can afford medical care, have developed a second system of charity care, which is somewhat less than second class. In the process we have disguised this kind of medical care by saying that charity patients receive outstanding medical care. There is a rather popular saying that the very rich and the very poor are the only ones who really receive decent medical treatment. This, like most folk sayings, is only half true because the poor do not receive adequate care—as can be demonstrated statistically or by actual observation of the kind of health care offered. The pesthouses and almshouses of an earlier era have been rebuilt or sometimes just renamed "county hospitals." Unlike governmental hospitals in most of the rest of the world, American county hospitals still utilize a means test to establish eligibility for care. Some private hospitals, particularly those maintained by religious or charitable organizations, also admit charity patients and apply similar means tests. These screening procedures psychologically separate the poor from the rest of the population, since a patient who qualifies has the stigma of knowing he passed the means test. Whatever his ethnic identity, the charity patient is also usually physically segregated from the paying customer, and he is treated with less deference than those who are able to afford private medicine.

The hospital is, however, only one aspect of health care, and nonwhite patients also receive less ambulatory care. Between 1965 and 1967 white patients averaged 4.5 physician visits a year (most of which were nonhospital visits) while nonwhite patients averaged 3.1 visits a year. Since people whose resources are limited are most likely to turn to the physician only when they are acutely ill, it was the preventive care and the early diagnosis and treatment that was most lacking. This lack of early diagnosis was revealed in a rather roundabout fashion in a recent report from the ongoing health interview survey carried out by the U.S. Public Health Service. Though it is generally known that nonwhite patients die earlier from a range of serious illnesses, and that they miss more days of work per year for serious illness (6.6 days compared to 5.5 for the white group), it was not realized that these people simply did not know how ill they were. When questioned as to whether anyone in their family had certain specific illnesses including arthritis, hypertension, heart trouble, ulcers, diabetes, or a vascular lesion, nonwhite patients were less likely to say yes than white were. Of the white patients, 51 percent reported that someone in their family had a specific chronic illness, but only 40 percent of the nonwhite people interviewed reported that a family member suffered from one of the conditions listed by the interviewer.[14] Since all the evidence, including autopsy records, indicate that poor people actually have more illnesses than the affluent, the underreporting of chronic illnesses in this study seems to be due to a lack of diagnosis. The ghetto resident is undoubtedly aware that he has some kind of "misery" but he cannot put the concise diagnostic label on it without the help of a physician. He probably does not even know that in many cases he could be cured or at least made more comfortable.

Discrimination

In addition to the problems faced by all poor people of any ethnic identity, nonwhite patients also in the past have been denied adequate health care because of discrimination or segregation, and though such discrimination is no longer quite so obvious, it undoubtedly exists. When Gunnar Myrdal made his famous pioneering study of the Negro in America, which was completed in 1942, he reported widespread medical discrimination and segregation. Segregation existed not only in the South but also in the North, though it was more open in the South. Some southern hospitals treated both white and black patients but segregated them, in inadequate and inferior wards, or refused to allow Negro doctors to treat their patients in such institutions. Some of the larger cities had all-Negro hospitals which, of course, had Negro doctors on their staffs. In the North and in the West the patterns varied; in some states hospitals were theoretically open to Negroes on equal terms with whites, but in other states the courts had upheld the rights of the proprietors to prohibit or to segregate as they pleased.[15]

Not only was there discrimination in admissions, there was also discrimination in staffing.[16] Though both of these subjects will be discussed later in this book, it is important to emphasize the disastrous effect they had on medical care for Negroes. A U.S. Government survey of hospitals in 1963 found that Negroes were still denied access or were segregated; in fact, many of the medical care facilities which received federal grants under the Hospital Survey and Construction Act of 1946 (popularly known as Hill-Burton) practiced discrimination and as late as 1962 a U.S. District Court found that private hospitals need not be subject to the equal protection clause of the Fourteenth Amendment.[17]

With the beginnings of Medicare in 1966 all participating hospitals were required to sign an affidavit of nondiscrimination, and some 92 percent of the nation's hospitals were certified as meeting this requirement. In large areas of the South, however, many hospitals refused to adopt the nondiscriminatory provision, and at least 200 hospitals stated that they would make no attempt to comply; this included all hospitals in blocks of counties in Mississippi, northern Louisiana, southern Alabama, southern Georgia, and eastern South Carolina and Virginia.[18] Some of these institutions have since signed so that the era of open segregation and discrimination in hospital care is now more or less ended, but subtle forms of discrimination continue to exist. Some hospital admission officers still segregate patients, but now lacking a particular section that is labeled "colored," they admit the patient and move him around if a white patient needs the bed next to him, or they force him to take a private room. Moreover, there are still white physicians who ask Negro patients to come to the back door so that they will not be seen by the other patients.

Folk Medicine

Partly because of the humiliation involved in back-door medical care, but also because of a lack of funds and a general mistrust of traditional practitioners, folk medicine has remained important in the urban ghettoes and in the rural South. Folk medicine is, of course, an aspect of any culture, but its importance varies among groups in society depending upon income, education, and even discrimination. In an investigation of the process by which prospective patients arrive at the physician's door, Eliot Freidson found that most people went through a kind of lay referral system. That is, they asked the advice of friends and relatives and tried to deal with their symptoms themselves before calling a physician.[19] For well-educated professional persons, this period of self-treatment was usually relatively brief, but for people whose socioeconomic status was low or who felt estranged from the available medical practitioners because of cultural differences, the lay referral system was expanded. Such patients exhausted all the home remedies known to family members, friends, and even neighborhood unlicensed practitioners before they were forced to turn to a doctor because of the continued seriousness of their illness.

The origins of Negro folk medicine are mixed; some are African while others more clearly seem to have developed in the rural South.[20] Some of the beliefs are purely magical while others have been empirically tested over generations and seem, upon investigation, to be rather logical and reasonable kinds of treatments. An example of the purely magical actions are such practices as putting a knife under the bed to cut the pain of labor and delivery, or the wearing of a variety of amulets and charms to ward off disease. The empirical procedures include massage, heat and baths for rheumatism, and the use of various herb teas and poultices for colds. Such practices not only give comfort but help sustain the patient through difficult times. The chief repository of folk remedies in the Negro community, as in many other societies, are the older women who have gained such wisdom through long experience. In today's Negro community the older woman may have worked in a hospital, although often in a menial job, or perhaps she just seems to have a knack for such healing. Middle-class Negroes, like middle-class Caucasians, tend to have deserted the full range of folk remedies as more professional health services have become available to them. To the extent, however, that discriminatory practices operate in preventing access to adequate medical care, even some educated people are motivated to turn to folk practitioners for advice.

The Culture of Poverty

Medical care for minorities quite obviously is a complex problem, and it is not only because of poverty and discrimination that there is a difference in health between black and white Americans. Public health professionals often complain that poor people, and particularly poor Negroes, do not take advantage of the preventive care that is available. The complaint of these workers has been demonstrated to be true in repeated studies. People whose socioeconomic status is low or who are nonwhite make less use of health facilities than other people, and the kind of service they are least likely to seek is preventive health care.[21] The reason for this low level of utilization of available health services seems to be at least partly psychological. Slavery, plus the generations of poverty and segregation, have left their mark upon Negroes. This is not surprising because, even when discrimination is not a factor, poverty can be debilitating to the spirit.

In attempts to explain further the reasons as to why some groups make less effective use of facilities than others, various methods of classifying the poor into groups have been developed. One of the simplest and most useful of these typologies is a dichotomy used by John Kosa.[22] Kosa suggested that there is an essential difference between acute and chronic poverty. By his definition the acutely poor are those who had lived much of their life with an adequate income, at least by the standards of their society, but then suddenly either become unemployed, or gradually became old and have to live in reduced circumstances. The acutely poor face severe problems of adjustment because they have to find ways of coping with their new status of being poor. They are more likely to attempt to find ways to modify their condition. On the other hand, the chronically poor have spent their whole lives in poverty or, as in the case of the Negro, poverty has often been a multigenerational phenomenon. The chronically poor, accustomed to poverty as they are, have developed a whole pattern of life for coping with their condition. This pattern, which the anthropologist Oscar Lewis called the culture of poverty, is passed on from one generation to another. Based on his studies in Mexico City, New York, and San Juan (Puerto Rico), Lewis argued that the culture of poverty transcends racial and national lines and that some of the traits that have been attributed to nationality groups are actually common to all people caught in this condition. The culture of poverty must of necessity exist inside of another more affluent culture because the perception of being poor depends partly on knowing that there are others who are not poor. This culture is marked by a low level of political power and participation in the decision-making aspects of the society. In the families he studied, Lewis also found a low marriage rate, a high rate of illegitimacy, and many families headed by women, all of which are also common characteristics among those American Negroes whose socioeconomic status is low.

It is the psychological characteristics of the culture of poverty which seem to be most important for health care. Lewis found that fatalism, helplessness, dependence, and feelings of inferiority were common. He also found that the time orientation tends to be concentrated on the present rather than the future as is the case with middle-class society. The problem of getting through a day is enough without trying to bother about planning for the future.[23]

Others, mostly sociologists, have described the negative outlook of the people of the slums in terms of alienation; the poor feel cut off from power to control their own lives, and have no hope for the future improvement in their condition. With such an outlook a future time orientation would be foolish, so most poor people try only to deal with the problems at hand. The middle-class orientation, on the other hand, is linked to a system of deferred gratification because such planning has paid off, but the man who lives on the edge of starvation or disaster has never learned the value of deferring so he does not save money or, in the case of health, does not seek preventive health care.

The importance of alienation in describing the negative outlook of the poor has been the subject of considerable empirical research. It was found in one study that mothers who felt socially isolated and believed that they lacked the power to control their own lives or those of their children were less likely to bring their children into the well-baby clinics than mothers who felt less powerless and less isolated from the supports of friends and family.[24] In another study it was found that the negative feelings of despair and alienation as measured by the anomie scale constructed by Leo Srole acted as barriers to mothers seeking prenatal care as well as immunizations for their children.[25] There is simple logic in these findings since it would seem that the person who feels that he has no control over what happens to him would not see the value in taking the necessary steps to obtain preventive health care; in his own mind his health would be controlled by fate or other outside forces rather than his own actions.

Following this line of reasoning a comprehensive study of the psychological barriers to preventive health care was done by one of the authors (B.B.). During the winter and spring of 1970-71 eight hundred mothers from the poor neighborhoods of East and South-Central Los Angeles were interviewed. Those with minority status, incomes below the poverty line, and meager education tended to have a much more negative outlook on life. They felt powerless, isolated, and hopeless. These feelings in turn were related to a low level of utilization of preventive health services for themselves and their children. This meant fewer check-ups, less dental care, fewer immunizations and less prenatal care. However, the most significant correlations were with the various indices of effective family planning. Family planning seemed almost impossible for the alienated black or Mexican-American woman from a poverty neighborhood, even when services were available at a near-by clinic.

Numerous previous studies have shown the correlation between effective family planning and socioeconomic status,[26] but alienation as a factor is just starting to be investigated.[27] Lee Rainwater pointed out that a sense of stability and trust in the future were essential preconditions for consistent family planning and since these conditions were not present among the poor, effective long-range planning is rare.[28] Race also is a factor. Negro women whose socioeconomic status is low have more difficulty with family planning than white women at a comparable level. In spite of the fact that the Negro women desired a limited number of children they ended up giving birth to more.[29] This emphasizes that although poverty itself is important in creating the negative feelings that deter planning and preventive behavior, segregation and discrimination magnify the effects of poverty. In a study of housing patterns done earlier by an author of this book it was found that segregation was a more important factor in creating feelings of alienation than simple poverty. Middle-class Negroes were studied so that poverty was not a current factor in their lives, although many of them had been poor in the past. Central to the findings was the fact that experience with segregated schools and a segregated life style was more strongly related to current feelings of powerlessness and hopelessness than past poverty. Unfortunately these feelings of alienation then in turn acted as barriers to integration so that segregation and alienation seem to relate to each other in a circular fashion.[30]

These findings do not necessarily contradict the idea that there is a culture of poverty transcending racial and national lines, but they do suggest that the experience of American Negroes with discrimination of various sorts may have added to their feelings of fatalism, hopelessness, and powerlessness. Since such subjective factors act as barriers to preventive health care, it seems obvious that it is necessary to have a multifaceted program to cure the inequalities now existing between white and nonwhite citizens in order to deal completely with the poor health of black Americans.

Obviously preventive health care is more important to some kinds of illnesses than others. We as yet can do little to prevent many of the degenerative processes associated with aging. However, an increasing number of contagious diseases can be prevented by immunization. In 1970, for example, there were several outbreaks of diphtheria in large urban areas which need not have occurred if immunizations had been available to all or if we could find a way of overcoming the powerlessness and hopelessness which keep the people of the ghettoes and barrios from bringing their children in for injections.

Perhaps the most obvious improvement would take place in the maternal mortality. In 1915 the mortality rate for nonwhite mothers of 105.6 per 1,000 births exceeded the rate for whites by 75 percent (60.0 per 1,000). Since that time the overall maternal death rate has fallen due to the improvements in the nature of hospitals and in medical and nursing knowledge. However, as the rates have fallen the gap between white and nonwhite mothers has grown until today it is 300 percent higher (7.2 per 1,000 births for the nonwhite and 2.2 per 1,000 for the white mothers).[31] To equalize the rates the whole nature of the health care delivery care system would have to be changed, although some statistical improvement undoubtedly could be made with the present system if ways could be found to encourage the nonwhite mother to seek more prenatal care.

One of the most obvious areas in which preventive medicine could be effectively applied is in the field of dentistry. Surprisingly, perhaps for hereditary reasons, Negroes suffer less from dental caries than do white Americans. The first indication of this was found by R. W. Hyde in his study of draft recruits in World War II, although his results have since been replicated. Only Chinese-Americans had fewer caries than American Negroes.[32] Negroes as a group, however, visit dentists much less than most other groups in American society, largely because dentistry is so expensive and is associated with middle-class status. In a sociological study of attitudes towards illness, E. L. Koos divided his sample into three socioeconomic groups: (I) business and professionals; (II) skilled and semiskilled workers, and (III) unskilled workers. Almost 95 percent of the Class I households reported they had a family dentist, but only 12.5 percent of the Class III families had established such a relationship. In fact 57 percent of the individuals in Class III and 9 percent of the individuals in Class II reported that they turned to dentists only to have a tooth extracted.[33] Koos' study is undoubtedly indicative of general attitudes towards dentists, and since so many Negroes are trapped in the culture of poverty, they get very little preventive dental care. Additional evidence for this assumption comes from the fact that Negroes have a much higher proportion of periodontal disease than whites, something which can be treated early by a dentist and often even prevented. In one study in which a scale ranging from zero to eight was used to rate the amount of periodontal disease the white population was given a score of 1.1 while the Negro population rated 1.6.[34]

Concluding Comments

In summary, it should be evident that the health problems faced by the large proportion of the Negro minority community are monumental. In part these difficulties can be understood through looking at the past history of the American Negro because this past has left its mark on today. Three variables seem most important in explaining the fact that mortality and morbidity rates are higher for Negroes: poverty, discrimination, and the social-psychological barriers which tend to keep people from using the services that are available. All three of these factors interact and reinforce each other just as poor health care interacts with and reinforces the other problems faced by black Americans.

Notes

1. For a moving account of some of the difficulties faced by the migrants read the novel *The Grapes of Wrath*, by John Steinbeck.
2. A popularized summary of some of these historical figures can be found in C. Eric Lincoln, *The Negro Pilgrimage in America* (New York: Bantam Books, 1967), p. 9.
3. E. Franklin Frazier, *Black Bourgeoisie* (New York: Collier Books, 1962), pp. 15-16.
4. E. Franklin Frazier, *The Negro Family in the United States* (Chicago: University of Chicago, 1939).
5. Melville J. Herskovits, *The Myth of the Negro Past* (Boston: Beacon Press, 1941), pp. 1 ff., and Melville J. Herskovits, *The New World Negro*, edited by Frances S. Herskovits (Bloomington: Indiana University Press, 1966).
6. See John Hope Franklin, *From Slavery to Freedom* (New York: A. A. Knopf, 1967), pp. 324-43, for further amplification.

7. Karl E. Taeuber and Alma F. Taeuber, *Negroes in Cities* (Chicago: Aldine Company, 1965), p. 14.
8. U.S. Department of Health, Education, and Welfare *Vital Statistics of the United States*, 1967, vol. II, *Mortality*, (Washington, D.C.: U.S. Government Printing Office, 1968), Table 5-6.
9. Mollie Orshansky, "Who Was Poor in 1966?" *Research and Statistics Note*, No. 23 (Washington, D.C.: U.S. Department of Health, Education and Welfare, 1967), Table 6.
10. Peter M. Blau and Otis Dudley Duncan, *The American Occupational Structure* (New York: John Wiley, 1967), pp. 207-242.
11. U.S. Department of Labor, *The Negro Family: The Case for National Action* (Washington, D.C.: U.S. Government Printing Office, 1965), p. 66.
12. "Watts: Everything Has Changed—and Nothing," *Newsweek* (Aug. 24, 1970), pp. 58-60; Paul Bullock, *Watts: The Aftermath* (New York: Grove Press, 1969).
13. U.S. Department of Health, Education, and Welfare, *Medical care, Health Status and Family Income*, United States, Vital and Health Statistics, Public Health Publication No. 1000, Series 10, No. 9, p. 6 (Washington, D.C.: U.S. Government Printing Office, 1964).
14. U.S. Department of Health, Education, and Welfare *Differentials in Health Characteristics by Color*, United States Vital and Health Statistics, July 1965-June 1967, Public Health Publication No. 1000, Series 10, No. 56, p. 5 (Washington, D.C.: U.S. Government Printing Office, 1969).
15. Gunnar Myrdal, with the assistance of Richard Sterner, and Arnold Rose, *An American Dilemma: The Negro Problem and American Democracy* (New York: Harper & Brothers, 1944), pp. 635-36.
16. Vern and Bonnie Bullough, *What Color Are Your Germs?* (Chicago: Committee To End Discrimination in Chicago Medical Institutions, 1955), and *The Untouchables* (Chicago: Committee Against Discrimination and the Southern Conference on Education, 1955).
17. *Civil Rights '63*, Report of the United States Commission on Civil Rights (Washington, D.C.: U.S. Government Printing Office, 1963), pp. 133-34.
18. Norman Dorsen, *Discrimination and Civil Rights* (Boston: Little, Brown and Company, 1969), p. 463, note 1.
19. Eliot Freidson, "Client Control and Medical Practice," *American Journal of Sociology*, 65 (1960), pp. 374-382.
20. Newbell Niles Puckett, *Folk Beliefs of the Southern Negro* (reprinted New York: Dover, 1969). This study, though a pioneering investigation when it was first published in 1926, would not meet today's standards of scholarship because it jumps from one time and period to another; nevertheless, it does contain considerable information.
21. Earl Loman Koos, *The Health of Regionville* (New York: Columbia University Press, 1954); George James, "Poverty and Public Health— New Outlooks: 1. Poverty as an Obstacle to Health Progress in Our Cities," *American Journal of Public Health*, 55 (November 1965), pp. 1757-1771; Leila C. Deasy, "Socio-Economic Status and Participation in the Poliomyelitis Vaccine Trial," *American Sociological Review*, 21 (April 1956), pp. 185-191; Elizabeth L. Watkins, "Low-Income Negro Mothers—Their Decision to Seek Prenatal Care," *American*

Journal of Public Health, 58 (April 1968), pp. 655-667; Nancy Milio, "Values, Social Class and Community Health Services," *Nursing Research*, 16 (Winter 1967), pp. 26-31.

22. John Kosa, "The Nature of Poverty," *Poverty and Health: A Sociological Analysis*, edited by John Kosa, Aaron Antonovsky, and Irving Kenneth Zola (Cambridge, Mass.: Harvard University Press, A Commonwealth Fund Book 1969), pp. 1-33.

23. Oscar Lewis, *La Vida: A Puerto Rican Family in the Culture of Poverty* (New York: Random House, 1965), pp. xlii-lii; Oscar Lewis, "The Culture of Poverty," *Scientific American* (October 1966), pp. 19-25. There are those who object to the concept of the culture of poverty; see for example Charles A. Valentine, *Culture and Poverty: Critique and Counter Proposals* (Chicago, University of Chicago Press, 1968).

24. Naomi M. Morris, Martha H. Hatch, and Sidney S. Chipman, "Alienation as a Deterrent to Well-Child Supervision," *American Journal of Public Health*, 56 (November 1966), pp. 1874-1882.

25. Helen Nakagawa, "Family Health Care Patterns and Anomie," an unpublished Ph.D. dissertation, University of California at Los Angeles, 1968.

26. P. K. Whelpton and Clyde V. Kiser, *Social and Psychological Factors Affecting Fertility*, vol. V (New York: Milbank Memorial Fund, 1958); Charles F. Westoff, Robert G. Potter, Jr., Philip C. Sagi, and Elliot Mishler, *Family Growth in Metropolitan America* (Princeton: Princeton University Press, 1961); Ronald Freedman, Pascal K. Whelpton, and Arthur A. Campbell, *Family Planning, Sterility and Population Growth* (New York: McGraw-Hill, 1959); Charles F. Westoff, Robert G. Potter, Jr., and Philip C. Sagi, *The Third Child* (Princeton: Princeton University Press, 1963).

27. H. Theodore Groat and Arthur G. Neal, "Social Psychological Correlates of Urban Fertility," *American Sociological Review*, 32 (December 1967), pp. 945-959.

28. Lee Rainwater, *And the Poor Get Children* (Chicago: Quadrangle Books, 1960).

29. Arthur A. Campbell, "Fertility and Family Planning Among Non-White Married Couples in the United States," *Eugenics Quarterly*, 12 (September 1961), pp. 124-131; Jack L. Roach, Lionel S. Lewis, and Murray A. Beauchamp, "The Effects of Race and Socio-Economic Status on Family Planning," *Journal of Health and Social Behavior*, 4 (March 1963), pp. 40-45.

30. Bonnie Bullough, "Alienation in the Ghetto," *American Journal of Sociology*, 72 (March 1967), pp. 469-78, and Bonnie Bullough, *Social-Psychological Barriers to Housing Desegregation* (Los Angeles: University of California, Graduate School of Business Administration, 1969).

31. Edith H. Anderson and Arthur J. Lesser, "Maternity Care in the United States: Gains and Gaps," *American Journal of Nursing*, 66 (July 1966), pp. 1539-1544.

32. R. W. Hyde, "Socioeconomic Aspects of Dental Caries," *New England Journal of Medicine*, 230 (1944), pp. 506-510. More recent studies have verified this finding. See Walter J. Pelton, John B. Dunbar, Russell S. McMillan, Palmi Moller, and Albert E. Wolff, *The Epidemiology of Oral Health* (Cambridge: Harvard University Press, 1969), p. 9, Table 1.7.

33. Earl Loman Koos, op. cit. pp. 118-125.
34. Pelton, Dunbar, *et al.*, *op. cit.*, Table 2.7. See also "Selected Dental Findings In Adults By Age, Race and Sex, United States, 1960-1962," Vital and Health Statistics, U.S. Department of Health, Education, and Welfare, Public Health Publication No. 1000, Series 11, No. 7 (Washington, D.C.: U.S. Government Printing Office, 1969).

4

The Spanish-Speaking Minority Groups

The fastest growing minority groups in the United States today are the Spanish-speaking peoples from various parts of the Western Hemisphere, particularly Mexico, Puerto Rico, and Cuba. Although characterized by a common language and grouped together for statistical purposes by their Spanish surnames, these three groups reflect quite different traditions. The largest of the nationality groups, and the one that has been in the United States the longest is the Mexican-Americans, or as some of the militants now term themselves, Chicanos.

Mexican-Americans

Most immigrants to the United States arrived by sea, but the Mexican-Americans simply moved northward. In fact, many of them lived in the southwestern part of the United States before it became part of this country or English-speaking pioneers moved westward. The closeness of the vast majority of Mexican-Americans to their homeland, and their unique treaty rights with

63

the United States tend to set them apart from most other immigrants.

The Mexican-American War, fought between 1846 and 1848, serves as the watershed for the history of Mexican-Americans in the United States. Under the treaty of Guadalupe Hidalgo, executed on February 2, 1848, Mexico ceded a vast territory including California, Arizona, New Mexico, Nevada, Utah, and much of Colorado, and also approved the prior annexation of Texas, previously a part of Mexico. The ceded lands represented one-half of the territory possessed by Mexico in 1821 when it had gained independence from Spain.

According to the provision of the treaty all citizens of Mexico who decided to remain within the ceded territory were to become citizens of the United States. It is estimated that as a result some 75,000 Spanish-speaking people became American citizens. The treaty also provided specific guarantees for the property and political rights of these Spanish-speaking Americans, who were given the right to retain their language, their religion, and their culture. No provision was made for the integration of the peoples as a group into American society, although the treaty did contain a promise of early statehood for the area. California, which had about 7,500 Spanish-speaking inhabitants, was quickly admitted into the Union, as was Nevada which had almost no Spanish-speaking residents. Texas, with some 5,000 Spanish Americans, was already a state. New Mexico with its 60,000 former Mexican nationals and Arizona with approximately 1,000 were much slower to receive statehood. One reason for the delay was the fact that neither of these future states had many Anglo-American citizens and American politicans were reluctant to grant full civil rights to a people they considered to be largely illiterate and of an "alien" culture. The effect of this attitude toward the indigenous Mexican-Americans was to retard assimilation and to encourage the survival of the Spanish cultural influence.

Though descendents of these Mexican nationals, as well as later immigrants from Mexico, have all been classified as Spanish-speaking Americans, the term at best is a very ambiguous one since Mexico itself was and is home to many different peoples. Citizens of Mexico can be descendents of European settlers (Spanish as well as others), or of the indigenous Indians, or any mixture thereof. In the American Southwest people with Spanish surnames come from a variety of backgrounds. The mixed nature of this heritage is evident from the city of Los Angeles, which prides itself on its Spanish founders. Of these founders and their wives, two were Spaniards, two were Negroes, nine were of mixed Negro-Spanish or Spanish-Indian backgrounds, nine were Indians, and one was Chinese. All, presumably except for the Chinese person, whose name is unknown, had Spanish names.

Today the border between Mexico and the United States is some two thousand miles long, most of it desolate and sparsely populated. Until the Border Patrol of the U.S. Immigration Service was established in 1924 the border could be and was crossed in either direction with comparative ease. Moreover, much of northern Mexico is geographically separated from southern Mexico by deserts, which meant that the natural market and supply centers for much of the area were in the United States, particularly in those areas which had formerly been part of Mexico. There is also considerable geographical similarity between the Southwest part of the United States and northern Mexico so that Mexicans who moved north felt more or less at home. Inevitably there has been considerable movement of Mexicans back and forth across the border, although no one knows for certain the total number of those who crossed over. It is known, however, that in the period before 1900 Mexican nationals played an important part in pioneering new techniques in the gold and silver mining industry in the Western and Pacific states, in the growth of the sugar beet industry, in the development of irrigation, and in the emergence of Texas as a leading cotton-growing state.

Generally speaking, however, the Southwestern part of the United States did not begin to grow very fast until the last decade of the 19th century. This growth has continued through most of the 20th century; much of it has been due to the availability of cheap labor, mostly Mexicans who moved northward in large numbers. In the period between 1900 and 1930 it is estimated that some 10 percent of the total population of Mexico, over a million migrants, crossed into the United States. The Mexican population of Texas, for example, rose from 70,981 in 1910 to 683,681 in 1930. It was Mexican labor which built the railroads, dug the irrigation ditches, picked the cotton, cleared the land, and ultimately built the highways opening up the Southwest. This meant that the massive wave of Mexican-American immigration coincided in large part with mass exodus to this country of the Russian, Slavic, and Italian immigrants, but the Mexican-Americans never were so isolated from their homeland as most other would-be citizens, since Mexico in most cases was never more than 150 miles away.

In fact, the overwhelming majority of the Mexican migrants settled down in a fan-shaped area stretching out from the Mexican border up past Los Angeles to Santa Barbara on the Pacific Ocean and stretching eastward and southward through San Antonio to Corpus Christi on the Gulf of Mexico. Even today most persons of Mexican descent live in this narrow belt of territory which includes parts of Texas, California, Arizona, New Mexico, and Colorado. There has been a remarkable continuity of Mexican family life and customs in this area, in part because most Mexicans who have come north first moved in with relatives. Today large numbers of Mexican-Americans in the southwest United States have relatives across the border, which means there is considerable movement back and forth between the two countries. The extent and concentration of this Mexican migration has tended to make the border rather indistinguishable with a heavy shading of Mexican-Americans near the border, thinning out as one travels north. This shading is on both sides of the borders since increasing numbers of people who are not Mexican-Americans have retired in Mexico or have winter homes in northern Mexico. Moreover, travel between Mexico and the United States is comparatively easy because the boundary is an imaginary line which is marked only by a barbed wire fence, or an easily forded river which often changes its channel. The lack of effective natural border barriers has led to many problems but it also has tended to lessen the hostility between Mexico and the United States. We do not have the kind of enmity that the Germans and the French who face each other across the Rhine have, but rather there is a sort of gradual fusion between two cultures and people with the Spanish-speaking Americans in the Southwest providing a kind of organic union with the culture and civilization of Mexico.[1]

Immigration from Mexico has tended to be in spurts, depending in large part upon the economic conditions in the United States. Much of it has been through contract labor, a term used to describe imported workers whose freedom is restricted by the terms of contractual relations. Though contract labor, except in the case of skilled or professional workers, has been outlawed in the United States since 1885, various legal ways have been found to circumvent the law. One of the largest loopholes appeared in the immigration law of 1917, which contained a provision allowing the Commissioner of Immigration and Naturalization to control and regulate the admission and return of otherwise inadmissible aliens applying for temporary admission. This meant that though contract labor was still outlawed, large numbers of Mexican nationals could be imported into the United States, providing the consent of the Commissioner was obtained. During and following World War I some 50,000 workers are known to have been recruited in Mexico, many of whom were sent to northern states as well as the fields and industries of the Southwest. Some of the Mexicans who earlier had crossed the border into the United States were also recruited for work in northern states. In 1923, for example, the National Tube Company, an affiliate of U.S. Steel, brought 1,300 Mexicans from Texas to work in its Lorain, Ohio, plant. In that same year Bethlehem Steel imported 1,000 workers from Mexico to work in its plants in Pennsylvania. The Mexican colony in Detroit had its beginnings in 1918 when several hundred Mexicans were brought to work in the automobile industry as student workers, and others from Mexico soon followed.

The bulk of Mexicans who came north, however, were recruited originally as farm laborers. The changing nature of farming in the United States, and the Depression of the 1930s created great difficulty. In fact, by 1937, machines had taken over 90 percent of the work involved in preparing, bedding, and cultivating the land to produce garden crops, and this meant that farm labor became ever more seasonal with the greatest demand coming at harvest time. As the Mexicans, many of whom now regarded themselves as Americans, lost their jobs, they attempted to organize and to strike. In the Southwest there were a number of Mexican-led strikes which generally failed. Failure was due in part to the fact that immigration authorities usually deported those workers who were not citizens, while others were intimidated by threats of violence. Moreover, in most of the strikes, Mexican workers stood alone since they were not affiliated with the rest of organized labor. The result was a mass exodus of Mexicans from the United States to Mexico, often aided and encouraged by various governmental agencies. In February 1931, for example, the County of Los Angeles shipped a whole trainload of its residents back to Mexico at a cost of some $77,249.29. Authorities estimated that the county still saved $347,468.41 in relief money. In 1932 more than 11,000 Mexican nationals were repatriated from Los Angeles alone.[2]

With the advent of World War II there was once again a demand for workers, and Mexico seemed to be an obvious source. In May 1942, the United States and Mexico agreed upon conditions under which Mexicans might be recruited to work in the United States. Imported workers were to be provided free transportation to and from their homes in Mexico, were to be paid subsistence in route, were not to be used to displace other workers or to lower wages or salary rates, and were to be provided with certain minimum working and living conditions. On September 29, 1942, the first shipment of 1,500 Mexican *braceros*, as they were called, arrived in Stockton, California. In 1945 alone, some 120,000 workers were recruited for agricultural employment in the United States, after which they were to return to Mexico. In addition another 80,000 workers were imported from Mexico to work on maintaining railroad lines. The farm labor importation program came to an end in 1947, but there was still a demand for low-paid agricultural employees, and this demand led to human smuggling rings. To curtail this, Congress in 1952 reviewed and revised the wartime legislation to allow workers to be imported under temporary work permits or visas. In fairly rapid succession nearly 500,000 workers were imported, the bulk of whom were from Mexico. Since that time there has been a gradual phasing out of most contract laborers, who were not only unpopular with organized labor but also with the domestic migratory farm workers who felt they were being used as strike breakers. Mexicans now enter legally under a general quota which covers all Western Hemisphere countries as immigrants, obtain work permits for temporary stay, or slip across the border illegally. Illegal immigrants can quickly lose themselves in the large ghettos, called barrios, of Spanish-speaking Americans.

In 1960 there were 3.5 million persons of Mexican ancestry in the five states of the Southwest, and this number has now been estimated at five million.[3] Since the change in the nature of agriculture, and the lessening demand for farm laborers, the majority of the Mexicans have come to settle in urban areas with the result that Los Angeles is second only to Mexico City in its total Mexican population. Like the Negroes, the Mexican-American is also segregated within the urban complex, although in most of the cities of the Southwest the housing patterns are not quite so rigidly segregated as those of Negroes. In Los Angeles, for example, there are great barrios which border the city on the east but there are also large numbers of Mexican-Americans scattered throughout the city. Since many people with Spanish surnames have achieved positions of power and influence in the Southwest, discrimination against Mexican-Americans tends to be far more subtle than that experienced by Negroes. However, most members of the Mexican-American minority are still poor and they still face a language barrier. Although the immigrant cannot advance to a position of influence in the outside world without learning English, it is possible to live a lifetime in the larger barrios without becoming fluent in English. This means that many of the children from the barrios who go to school are bilingual, speaking Spanish at home and English at school. This tends to discourage all but the most dedicated students from continuing their schooling. More-over, the fact that many of the Mexicans are in this country illegally makes the Mexican-American worker more exploitable because an unscrupulous employer can hire an illegal immigrant and use the threat of exposure over him or his friends or relatives as a power tool in order to pay him less than minimum wages or to avoid enforcing safety rules.

The peasant Mexican culture, from which most of the Mexican-Americans derived, also tends to work against easy assimilation into the Anglo-American middle-class culture. Also, Mexico and the United States have, with few exceptions, enjoyed fairly peaceful relationships for over a century and this has meant that the Mexicans did not have to choose between their mother country and the United States as some German-Americans felt they had to do in World War I. This has made it possible for large numbers of Mexican-Americans to live together geographically in the United States but intellectually and emotionally in the local Mexican tradition. Moreover, Mexico at least in the period before World War I, was a very poor country with society so organized that the sense of enterprise, thrift, and initiative highly valued by Americans was not encouraged. The patron system of land tenure in Mexico was not unlike the southern plantation system, which meant that the workers or peons were virtually powerless. In societies of this type money is meaningless, trade is limited, and division of labor is either simple or almost nonexistent. In Mexico native folk practices were interwoven with Catholic Church ritual. Inevitably the Mexican peon could rather easily become confused and demoralized in the American city. Unfortunately these culturally conditioned traits have often been interpreted as racial or biological. The Mexican stereotype is usually one of extremes, either lawless and violent, or lacking in ambition and lazy. As a defense against these stereotypes and discrimination in-group feeling has developed, while on the other hand those Mexicans who have managed to achieve in American society often cut themselves off from their countrymen by emphasizing that they are Spanish instead of facing up to the cultural stereotype of being Mexican.

Puerto Ricans

Puerto Rico was occupied by the United States in 1898 during the Spanish-American War and was ceded to this country as part of the treaty with Spain. Though our stated intention had been to provide revenues and civil government only on a temporary basis, annexation was soon followed by American investment which revolutionized the production of sugar and changed the nature of farming on the island. In 1917 the Organic Act, sometimes called the Jones Act, admitted all Puerto Ricans to American citizenship except those who petitioned to retain their former political status. Puerto Rico itself was recognized as an "organized but unincorporated territory." Jurisdiction over the territory was in the hands of the War Department until 1934 when it was transferred to the Interior Department, but it was not until 1947 that the Puerto Ricans could elect their own governor. In 1950 Congress passed legislation allowing Puerto Rico to become a Commonwealth and in 1952 the Commonwealth of Puerto Rico was established. This meant that Puerto Rico was a self-governing political unit voluntarily associated with the United States whose inhabitants were American citizens.

United States annexation changed the economic organization of the island, while the introduction of American medical techniques and sanitary improvements lowered the death rate. The result was a rapid growth in population which was not matched by an increase of jobs. The population of 953,243 in 1899 had grown to 2,210,703 by 1950, in spite of large-scale migration to the United States. The island's current population density of more than 700 people per square mile makes it one of the most densely populated areas of the world. From 1901 to 1960 Puerto Rico's death rate dropped from 36.7 per 1,000 to a subnormal 6.7, a figure lower than that recorded in the United States. The birth rate, however, declined at a much slower rate, from 43.2 in 1947 to 31.5 in 1960. Though vast strides were made in economic progress, particularly in the last few decades which saw the annual per capita income of $120 in 1940 rise to $740 in 1963, the median income is still far below that of any American state. Inevitably, large numbers of islanders migrated to the United States for work. During the 1950s some 50,000 people a year left the island, a rate which has somewhat declined in recent years, in part because many older people are now returning. There is still, nonetheless, a consistent outpouring of residents into the United States.[4]

Before 1920 there were only an estimated 15,000 Puerto Ricans residing in the United States. Once the Puerto Ricans were given citizenship, however, their status changed from immigrant to migrant, and the numbers rapidly increased. In the decade 1921-1930, some 52,774 settled on the mainland; 1931-1940, 69,967; 1941-1950, 226,110; 1951-1960, 615,384. It is estimated that there are now more than one million Puerto Ricans living in the United States, some 600,000 of them in New York City.[5] Unlike early settlers, the Puerto Ricans came by air, and the comparative ease with which they can migrate has encouraged them to consider themselves only as temporary residents. Like the Mexican-Americans of the Southwest, there is also considerable two-way traffic between the island and the mainland.

Puerto Ricans are of mixed racial origins. The original Spanish conquest was so devastating that the Indian population was virtually wiped out. Most of the present inhabitants are descendants of the Spanish and their Negro slaves, with only a slight Indian mixture. In the 1960 census return approximately 20 percent of the island population was classified as nonwhite. There is, however, a wide variation in skin color among the population and although there is no formal segregation or discrimination based upon skin color there is informal prejudice against the darker members of society, particularly if their socioeconomic status is also low. Nonetheless, in New York City and other urban centers to which they have migrated this comparative lack of prejudice and identity related to skin color has created considerable controversy between Puerto Ricans and Negroes. Negroes expected the dark Puerto Ricans to give support to the civil rights and black power movements, but in the past these people have been much more likely to identify with their light-skinned cousins from Puerto Rico than with American Negroes.

Since Puerto Ricans, in spite of intense efforts, still have low educational levels in Puerto Rico, and are the newest migrants to the eastern cities, they also tend to be the poorest. They have inherited the most deteriorated slum areas, many moving into formerly black areas which the upwardly mobile Negroes were happy to leave behind. The newly arrived workers also tend to find jobs as laborers or machine operators, which in New York usually means they work in the garment industry. Although there are as yet few second-generation Puerto Ricans resident on the continent, some intergenerational upward mobility has been noted. A 1960 comparison of first- and second-generation migrants indicated that while only 15 percent of the first-generation workers held white collar jobs, 31 percent of the second-generation workers were in white collar occupations. In spite of this statistical progress, however, the overwhelming majority of Puerto Ricans in this country hold very low-level jobs, and are susceptible to being laid off as soon as the rate of unemployment rises.

Cubans

Cuba was long closely tied economically to the United States, and in the past some analysts spoke of it as being essentially an economic dependency of the United States. The United States had originally become involved in the war with Spain largely as a result of Cuba's efforts to free itself, and though we recognized the independence of Cuba we were ceded a large naval base, Guantanamo Bay, in Cuba itself. The United States also reserved the right to intervene militarily in Cuba whenever it felt Cuban independence was threatened. American investment soon dominated Cuba, which in turn led to a considerable movement of Cubans to the United States. Even before the Spanish-American War the cigar industry in Key West and Tampa had been founded by Cuban refugees. By 1960 the population of Cuban stock in the United States totalled 124,416 persons of whom 116,354 were classified as white and 8,062 nonwhite. It is interesting to note that although Negroes comprised an estimated 25 percent of the Cuban population, only about 6.5 percent of the Cubans coming to the United States before the Castro takeover were classed as Negroes. Most of the early Cuban immigrants settled in Florida and New York—although New Jersey, Illinois, and California also had large numbers of Cubans.

The nature of this Cuban immigration changed radically when Fidel Castro overthrew the dictatorship of Fulgenico Batista at the beginning of 1959. Many of Batista's followers fled to the United States, and soon afterwards Castro launched an intensive propaganda campaign blaming many of the ills of his country on Americans. By the end of 1960, in retaliation for the United States elimination of the Cuban sugar import quota, Castro nationalized United States investments in Cuba—which amounted to more than one billion dollars. The United States broke diplomatic relations with Cuba at the beginning of 1961, and relations between the two countries have not been much improved since. An increasing number of Cubans sought refuge in the United States as Castro tightened his control on the country and adopted a program of encouraging those who did not agree with him to leave. There were regularly scheduled air flights from Cuba to Miami from the end of 1959 to October 1962, when they were discontinued during the missile crisis. A second large-scale exodus of Cubans began late in 1965 when the United States and Cuba agreed to allow special flights from Havana to Miami. As self-imposed political exiles, the Cubans were admitted under special refugee quotas. Most of them probably never intended to settle in the United States permanently, but rather to go back to Cuba as soon as Castro was overthrown. For a time, in fact, many of them were deeply involved in revolutionary activities designed to overthrow Castro. With the passage of time, however, more and more of them have begun to settle down and begin the process of becoming American citizens. In the first great exodus from Cuba between 1959 and 1962 it is estimated that nearly a quarter of a million refugees arrived in the United States, with a high point of 3,000 a week at Miami airport just before the Cuban missile crisis.[6] The second wave of refugees has been nearly as large.

Since most of the refugees were forced to leave money and possessions behind them as a condition for exit from Cuba, they often arrived only with the clothes on their backs. In spite of this, the Cubans differed from most other past migrants to these shores, and particularly from the Mexican-Americans and the Puerto Ricans in both their educational levels and their sophistication. Though there are refugees from all classes of pre-Castro Cuban society, from illiterate peasants to millionaires, a disproportionate number came from the middle and upper strata of society. The overwhelming majority of them, in fact, can be classified as professional, semiprofessional, managerial, white collar, or as skilled workers. This means that once the trauma of relocation was over, the vast majority of them were able to earn adequate or even high-level incomes and did not suffer from the long-term, poverty-related health problems. Undoubtedly, however, the loss in status was extremely painful, and the problems of adjusting to another language meant added burdens, but most of the Cubans adjusted fairly rapidly. Many of the professionals had to undergo new training or gain additional experience to qualify for American licensure, and some—such as lawyers—had to find a new occupation because Cuban law has little in common with American.

The greatest health problems occurred in Florida as the refugees first landed. Control of epidemics is always a problem when large numbers of people are moved into temporary and crowded quarters, and this problem was complicated by the communication barriers. Eventually Cuban nurses were hired as aides by the Miami health department until they qualified for American licensure and they proved remarkably effective in bridging the health information gap. Perhaps the most pressing problem were the more than 13,000 unaccompanied children who were sent by frightened parents who were not at all sure that they themselves would ever be able to join them. Most of these parents eventually did leave Cuba and reestablished their families, but for a time the placement of the children and the problem of helping them to adjust to the loneliness and new surroundings was an overwhelming task for the workers in Miami. It should be added that the federal government itself assumed a greater burden for these immigrants to American shores than for any other group, and in fact up to 1967 the government had spent more than 200 million dollars in assisting Cubans to retrain and relocate, an average of about $1,000 per adult Cuban.[7]

Health Problems of Mexican-Americans

Since Mexican-Americans are lumped together with other whites in official records, comparisons of their mortality and morbidity rates with those of other groups are difficult. It is not, however, impossible. There have been some studies of mortality rates which use the Spanish surname as a category, and these studies suggest that Mexican-Americans share the poverty-related health problems that are the main cause of poor health among Negroes. A study of mortality rates conducted in Colorado indicated that the people with Spanish surnames were much more likely to die of rheumatic fever, pneumonia, and influenza than were members of the Anglo population. Since the timely administration of antibiotics for streptococcic infections can prevent rheumatic fever from ever developing while the mortality rate for pneumonia and influenza can be lessened by early treatment, it seems obvious that these death rates are clearly related to a lack of adequate medical care.

The Colorado study also found that neonatal deaths were three times as high among the Spanish-surname group as among Anglos, reflecting not only less adequate conditions at and following delivery but also a lack of prenatal care as well as the poor general nutrition and health of the mother. Fatal accidents were also a major cause of death among members of the Spanish-surname population, and although lack of medical care may again be implicated here, the Colorado commission which sponsored the study believed that the use of old automobiles and unsafe equipment was the most important factor in explaining this finding.[8]

The city of San Antonio annually publishes statistics which allow comparisons to be made among the Mexican-American, white, and nonwhite populations. In general these tabulations support the findings of the Colorado study; respiratory diseases were a major cause of death and infant mortality rates are high. In addition, in San Antonio there is a noticeably high fatality rate from diabetes among both the nonwhite and Mexican-American population. Although the fatality rate is again partly due to a lack of medical care, this is not the whole cause of the differential rate because other studies have shown that the diabetes morbidity rate is also higher among these two ethnic groups than it is among the population in general.[9] More complete explanations for these differences await basic research into genetic factors as well as the effects of the high-starch diet which so often accompanies poverty.

It is interesting to note that Mexican-Americans are much less likely to die of neoplasms, vascular diseases, and heart disease than other Americans. These diseases, commonly associated with aging, are much less common among all poverty populations, undoubtedly because of their earlier age of death from other causes. There is, however, some indication that the life styles associated with affluence may help cause heart and vascular diseases, and affluence is not yet a problem for the Mexican-Americans as a group.

In talking to the residents of the barrios one gathers that discrimination in obtaining health care is not so important to them as it is to Negroes, perhaps because discrimination is overshadowed by the problems associated with the language barrier and other aspects of the cultural barrier separating Mexican-Americans from Anglos. The monolingual Spanish-speaking patient finds a visit to an English-speaking physician or an American hospital frightening and often not particularly fruitful. Unless he takes a bilingual friend with him as an interpreter the exchange of information is apt to be meager because few health professionals in the Southwest are Spanish-speaking. The East Los Angeles Health Task Force, a community-based organization which had temporary funding from the Office of Economic Opportunity gathered information about the experiences of barrios residents when they confronted the Anglo health care system. They reported that a frightened old man watched a young Anglo physician give him penicillin in spite of the fact that he and his excited family were sure he was allergic to the drug and tried to tell this to the doctor who did not understand them. There are numerous stories of patients who were taken to surgery who did not know they were going to be operated on, as well as tales about people who were merely being transferred from one ward or area to another and thought they were going to surgery. After considerable agitation the Health Task Force was able to convince Los Angeles County Hospital that more Spanish-speaking nurses' aides and attendants should be hired so that interpreters would be available not only to assist with taking the patients' history but also to explain the hospital procedures to the patients.

Puerto Rican Health

Puerto Ricans are as concentrated on the Eastern Seaboard as Mexican-Americans are in the Southwest. The climate of New York City, however, is radically different from that of Puerto Rico, so that these people must adjust to a more radical change in living conditions than the Mexican-Americans in the Southwest. Population is also much more concentrated in the eastern part of the United States than in the western, so that overcrowding and unsanitary conditions lead to additional health problems. Since they are new migrants, the Puerto Ricans tend to settle in the most depressed housing areas where their residences are often heavily infested with rats. The New York City Department of Health between 1947 and 1953 reported an average of 500 cases of rat bites each year, an extremely high percentage of them among Puerto Rican families.[10]

Tuberculosis was long endemic in Puerto Rico and until fairly recently Puerto Rico had a higher death rate from tuberculosis than any country that gathers statistics. This susceptibility to tuberculosis is often increased by poor, overcrowded housing conditions in the United States, as well as by deficient knowledge about health care and sanitation practices. Between 1949 and 1951 there were 474 reported cases of tuberculosis per

100,000 Puerto Rican residents.[11] Earlier (in the 1930s) Puerto Ricans living in New York had a higher mortality rate from tuberculosis than did those Puerto Ricans who remained on the island.[12] In a 1958 study of some 80 Puerto Rican families living in New York City, nine patients in six of the families were undergoing treatment for tuberculosis.[13]

Puerto Ricans also suffer from a variety of parasitic diseases including dysentery; malaria; filariasis (caused by a small worm which lives in the lymphatics of the body and is spread by the mosquito); schistosomiasis mansoni (dependent upon a snail carrier), which attacks the liver; and hookworm (also found in the American South). The New York City Health Department has stated that the generally poor health conditions of large numbers of Puerto Ricans was largely due to the presence of these parasites.[14]

Influencing the general health of the Puerto Rican migrants is widespread malnutrition. The chief articles of food on the island for the poorer people are rice and beans, with the beans serving as the main source of protein. Puerto Ricans eat few green or leafy vegetables, and only rarely do they use milk and eggs. Bread is also not generally used in all parts of the island. To this basic starch diet, the Puerto Rican adds cheap fats, usually lard or olive oil, in liberal quantities. Consequently internal disorders are widespread. When the Puerto Rican is transplanted to New York, the deficiency in his diet is made even worse by the relative lack of sunshine.

The effect of migration upon health was demonstrated in a New York City study which found that 20 percent of a sample of 216 migrants were hospitalized within their first year after leaving Puerto Rico.[15] In the years following the first one, there tended to be a decline in hospitalization. The reasons for this are not entirely clear. It might be that those suffering from chronic diseases prior to migration are apt to seek treatment soon after arrival; in fact, a few of them seem to have been sent north by their doctors or their families for treatment of a specific illness. The trauma of moving itself might also tend to aggravate long-standing illnesses. Separation from home and family can cause a painful adjustment as well as some practical difficulties. Since the family pattern in both Mexico and Puerto Rico tends to be extended, the individual can call on and expect help from many relatives in times of illness or other crises. Inevitably, moving to the United States breaks up some of these units and although people may eventually reestablish the extended family pattern by helping relatives to move or by seeking out relatives who are already here, this often takes time, so that new migrants are forced to turn to clinics or hospitals for care which would have been available from relatives in their old environment.

The stress of moving is also further complicated by other family problems. Consensual unions are common in Puerto Rico,[16] but many of these unions are fairly stable so that they are for most practical purposes similar to the more formal union of marriage. However, under the impact of urbanization and migration the informal arrangements tend to break down[17] and the single man and woman are left alone to cope with the new environment, or women are left as heads of households. For a woman who has grown up expecting help from all of her female relatives as well as support from her husband, such a desertion can be overwhelming. For a man who has always been surrounded by relatives the new-found freedom may spell loneliness.

Health Care Institutions

Inevitably the first- or second-generation Mexican-American as well as the recent Puerto Rican immigrant faces the Anglo health care institutions with a certain amount of suspicion. One of the difficulties in treating tuberculosis among both of these groups has been the people's fear of the hospital; rather than go for hospitalization many people deny they have the disease until the case is very advanced.[18] Although physicians in Mexico have high standards, they are mainly confined to urban middle-class areas. The primary source of medical care in most Mexican villages as well as in the poorer sections of the cities is folk medical practitioners whose knowledge is based upon an elaborate and well-developed system of beliefs acquired outside of any regular educational institution. Though upper-middle-class Mexican-Americans, as well as the more Americanized person in the lower-income groups, have abandoned much of the folk medical practices, the newly arrived and the poor of the barrios usually favor the folk system over American scientific medicine. Often they divide diseases into two categories, consulting a folk practitioner for the traditional diseases but an Anglo doctor for "Anglo diseases." In an interview study of Mexican-American women living in a public housing project, it was found that the overwhelming majority knew about and used the folk system of diagnosis and therapy for at least part of their care.[19]

The major folk practitioner in the Mexican-American community is the *curandero* (*curandera* in the case of a woman) who not only has acquired considerable empirical knowledge but also possesses the charismatic qualities associated with the more spiritual aspects of the role. A good *curandero* shows great warmth and concern for both the patient and his family. He offers advice, gives treatment, but asks for no fee. Special prayers are often a part of his therapy. If the treatment proves successful the family is expected to give him an offering but if he fails nothing is expected. This means that the *curandero*, because he knows no fee will be forthcoming, will often refuse to treat a patient who from previous experience he knows he cannot cure or who he thinks has a bad prognosis. In these cases the family turns to the Anglo doctor or hospital. The implication of this is not lost upon the patient who tends to associate hospitalization and the American doctor with a fear of death or serious disability or otherwise he could have been cured by the *curandero*.

The *curandero* is not the only folk practitioner; usually before he is sought out home remedies will have been tried and a neighborhood *señora* (older woman) will have been consulted. Actually the line between the *señora* and the *curandera* is not a clear one because older women usually start out helping their friends and family during times of illness, and if they gain a reputation for success they then become known as healers. A male healer may start as a *sovador* who specializes in giving massages, although from the beginning he may use the more general term of *curandero*. The *partera* or midwife is also an important practitioner in Mexico, but to a lesser extent in the United States where hospital deliveries are more common.[20] The cultural acceptance of the *partera*, who is always a woman, still influences the attitudes of the Mexican-American woman who has been accustomed to think that the female reproductive process should be a private matter between women. Male obstetricians, groups of medical students, and the matter-of-fact attitudes of the hospital and clinic personnel often prove to be traumatic in such cases. This tends to act as a further barrier to a woman's seeking prenatal care or accepting contraceptives.

The *curandero* also exists in the Puerto Rican community, although the role is not so well institutionalized. There are a variety of spiritualists in Spanish Harlem who trace their healing arts back to cults imported not only from Puerto Rico but also from other Caribbean islands.[21] These spiritualists emphasize healing through religious or magical ceremonies, potions, and amulets rather than through empirical methods. There are also a variety of herbs and charms available which the layman can buy and use at home without consulting any practitioner. Although very often an older woman who has accumulated knowledge of these herbs and other home remedies will be consulted by her family or friends, she seldom takes this calling as an occupational role as her counterpart in the Mexican-American community might do.

Folk Diseases

Some of the diseases recognized by the various folk practitioners are more or less the standard diagnoses recognized by the more scientific medical community. There are, however, other kinds of illnesses which fit into an independent folk system of belief and practice, and it is for this group of diagnoses that the *curandero* is most likely to be consulted. Various researchers have worked out systems to classify or group these folk diseases. Margaret Clark, who did an in-depth study of the health beliefs and practices of one Mexican-American community, could fit most of them into four categories: (1) diseases of hot and cold imbalance, (2) dislocations of internal organs, (3) illnesses of magical origin, and (4) illnesses of emotional origin.[22] The hot and cold theory of illness has been traced back to ancient Greek theories which held that the healthy man was maintained in a balance between four humours (phlegm, blood, black bile, and yellow bile). Some of these humours were thought to be disproportionately hot while others were cold; an imbalance between the various essences caused illness. This body of medical theory was brought to the new world by the 16th century Spanish explorers and eventually diffused throughout Mexico. In the process the theory was somewhat altered and the original idea of the four humours was reduced to a dichotomy between hot and cold.[23]

Illness is thought to be caused by a disequilibrium which can be the result of a dietary imbalance or exposure. Usually a dietary regimen or herbs are prescribed to cure the imbalance. Whether a food used in this treatment is classified as hot or cold is not necessarily related to its actual temperature; ice, for example, is considered hot because it burns the mouth. That such foods as chili peppers and onion are classified as hot seems quite logical, but the classification of tomatoes, citrus fruits, cucumbers, and chicken as cold is less apparent to the outsider, and the fact that white beans are considered hot while red beans are called cold carries no clue to the uninitiated. It is apparent that the *curandero* must absorb a large body of knowledge in order to master the whole system. Because of the complexity of the system, the average individual usually does not know all of the classifications, and turns to the *curandero* for advice. Symptoms of imbalance include head colds, stomach upsets, and general malaise. Infants are thought to be particularly susceptible to "cold stomach," which means that dedicated believers in this system do not give cold foods, including citrus fruits, to their infants in spite of the exhortations of public health nurses. Expectant mothers are often cautious about eating too many foods which are classified as hot because it is believed this will cause their babies to have diaper rashes when they are born.

A common folk illness which is only tenuously related to the hot and cold theory is *empacho*. The symptoms of *empacho*— including a swollen abdomen, diarrhea, vomiting, and fever—are attributed to a *bolita* or small ball of food which is caught in the stomach. Sometimes massage or manipulation are used to dislodge the lump although at other times a dietary regimen is prescribed as it is for ailments caused by a hot and cold imbalance. If the *curandero* decides a special diet is necessary he will usually curtail the intake of cheese, bananas, eggs, and soft bread because it is believed that these foods have a tendency to form a *bolita*.[24] At other times a purgative is advised to clean out the stomach.[25]

Mollera ciada, or fallen fontanel, is the most common type of organ displacement. It is usually attributed to a too-sudden withdrawal of the nipple from the infant's mouth.[26] Symptoms of the ailment include diarrhea and vomiting. It is interesting that in folk medicine the cause and effect are often reversed from that of scientific medicine. In this case the severe dehydration which accompanies infant diarrhea is taken as evidence for a depressed fontanel. Dehydration can be fatal unless the diarrhea is checked and enough oral or parenteral fluids are given, but the folk practitioner does not realize this and the methods he tries are not really effective. He usually relies on topical remedies or he may hold the infant up by his heels over a basin of water to try to get the fontanel to resume its normal appearance. The fact that *mollera ciada* is such a well-known ailment is testimony to the fact that severe diarrhea is still common among infants in the Mexican-American community and it is still a leading cause of the high infant mortality rate.[27]

A less common ailment attributed to a misplaced organ is that of infertility, which is sometimes explained as being due to a fallen uterus. Barrenness is a cause of great sadness because marriage and family are such important aspects of the culture, and women who are mothers are the most highly respected. Barrenness is also regarded as a threat to the male since a man is measured by his *machismo* or manliness, including the ability to produce children.[28] The *curandero* may attempt to treat the infertility with religious and magical cures as well as massage.

Diseases of purely magical origin include those attributed to the evil eye (*mal ojo*) and to bad air (*mal aire*). A folk belief in the evil eye as a cause of illness seems to be almost world-wide in scope so that any health practitioner who is willing to step outside of the confines of the modern medical center and to communicate with people about their beliefs is likely to run into the concept of the evil eye. In Italy and other parts of Europe, religious medals may be worn to ward off the evil eye. In an unpublished study of hospitalized Egyptian infants done by the authors in 1966, it was found that approximately half of the mothers interviewed felt that their infants' illnesses had been caused by the "one with the evil eye." The women explained that the handsome, healthy male babies were the ones who were particularly vulnerable to this type of spell because they were the ones who were most likely to be the objects of envy from living persons as well as from free-floating evil spirits. Similarly, the unsophisticated Mexican-American mother may believe that when someone, particularly a woman, admires her infant but fails to touch him the baby will develop symptoms of *mal ojo* including fitful crying, wakefulness, diarrhea, vomiting, and fever. If the person who admires the child touches him the spell will be broken and no illness occurs. Unfortunately social workers and nurses are sometimes blamed for casting the spell because they unwittingly admire infants in this manner. Once the symptoms of *mal ojo* develop in either a child or an adult, the victim can be treated only by magical means.

Mal aire (bad air) as a cause of illness is not so well known throughout the world as the evil eye, although many peoples believe in vague types of airborne spirits which cause illness. Symptoms of *mal aire* can include facial paralysis, convulsions, or other frightening symptoms. The *curandero* may treat the disease with massage and counter-spells.

Strong emotions and emotional trauma are recognized throughout Latin America as a cause of illness. The folk practitioners and the medical profession are actually in substantial agreement in this regard, although they do not use the same diagnostic labels. In the American Southwest the two most common emotional illnesses are *susto* (fright) and *bilis* (anger). *Susto* is believed to occur most often in children, although no age is immune because *susto* seems to be broadly defined to include much more than what we would call fright; almost any traumatic emotional illness can be the cause of *susto*. Ritual prayers are a common treatment of *susto*, although they may be combined with use of herbal remedies. In such cases the *curandero* may also try to manipulate the physical and psychological environment of the patient in order to lessen the emotional stress, although he undoubtedly would not explain his actions in these terms. *Bilis* is more often a disease confined to adults. It is manifested by nervousness and emotional upset as well as the physiological symptoms of the type which psychologists and psychiatrists generally link with anxiety. Herbs and emotional support are used in its treatment.[29]

There is also a special folk diagnosis of an emotional illness which is recognized by the Puerto Ricans, an illness called *ataque*. It seems to be particularly widespread among lower-socioeconomic groups and represents a popular and conventional reaction to overwhelming catastrophe. Men and women appear to be equally susceptible. The episodes begin quite suddenly, usually without warning either to the spectators (a necessary part of the disease) or the patient. The patient sometimes utters a short cry or scream before sliding to the ground. Shortly after falling to the ground, or at the same time, he begins moving his arms and legs in a kind of coordinated fashion. These movements seem purposeful, and include beating the fists on the floor, striking out at persons nearby, or banging the head on the floor. Foaming at the mouth is common, but usually there is no incontinence or tongue biting as there would be in epilepsy. The attack usually ceases abruptly, with the individual resuming what he was doing before with little effect. During the *ataque* no special change in pulse, blood pressure, or neurological signs have been noted by attending physicians. The *ataque* usually lasts for 5 to 10 minutes, but may go on for hours, and some have continued for four days.[30] *Ataques* may occur once in a lifetime or become a continuing pattern of reaction in particular individuals.

It is worthy of comment that although there are accounts of successful collaboration between Western psychiatrists and Yorubu witch doctors in Nigeria, there does not seem to have been much collaboration between American health practitioners and Spanish folk healers. Anglo health workers tend either to ignore the folk beliefs and practices or try to "educate" their patients by deprecating the folk practitioners. Since available information suggests that the folk methods are often effective, it might well be that a creative cooperation between the two groups would improve the delivery of health services. The most obvious effectiveness of the folk practitioner seems to be in the field of mental illness. E. Gartly Jaco reported in 1959 that, in Texas, psychoses among the Spanish-surname population was less than among Anglos or among nonwhites.[31] Since that time there is evidence that the incidence of mental illness among the younger Mexican-American population is rising, and it may be that Jaco's findings were somewhat biased because there were few Mexican-Americans in publicly supported facilities.[32] Still, all the evidence to date gives strength to the idea that the emotional support given both by the extended family and the folk practitioners is at least as effective if not more effective in preventing mental health problems than the help available to the rest of the population whose socioeconomic status is equally low and who lack such practitioners.

Cooperation could be even more helpful in attempting to eliminate the delays when folk medicine is clearly inadequate for saving lives, as is the case with infant diarrhea. If some sort of mutual agreement could be worked out, the professional health worker would not need to insist on wooing the patient away from the folk healer in all cases; moreover, the mainstream medical practitioner could be more effective in the struggle to upgrade health if they could adopt some of the personal warmth and appearance of concern which the *curandero* has. All one needs to do is contrast the hospital admissions officer whose hand is out for cash or an insurance card before any treatment can be given with the *curandero* who says no payment is necessary unless he is successful. It is true that the *curandero* uses informal pressures to obtain his fees but he is much more subtle and less demanding than the fee-for-service system which characterizes Anglo medicine.

Closer working relationships with the folk practitioners, knowledge about the culture, and understanding of the individual patient could help the health worker deliver more useful care. Often the very definitions of health and illness differ between the professional and patient. In one study of these perceptions it was found that Mexican-American villagers in Colorado and New Mexico felt that if a man was not emaciated or in pain and could perform his work role adequately he was well and had no need for medical care.[33] The professional who holds a preventive orientation to illness may value health care for the well person in the form of immunizations and early treatment of illness before it is debilitating. Such workers would feel less frustrated if they realized that this difference in outlook exists to a certain extent among all poor people because a preventive health outlook correlates with an ability to control the future, and that poverty makes such control impossible. What the professional needs to do is make preventive services seem more reasonable to the patient by integrating them with the acute care which the patient realizes he needs. The practitioners would thus demonstrate that they are willing to do their share to bridge the gap which exists between the health care professionals and the members of these Spanish-speaking subcultures.

Notes

1. Carey McWilliams, *North From Mexico: The Spanish-Speaking People of the United States* (reprinted, New York: Greenwood Press, 1968), p. 62.
2. *Ibid.*, p. 193.
3. Ernesto Galarza, Herman Gallegos, and Julian Samora, *Mexican-Americans in the Southwest* (Santa Barbara: McNally & Loftin, in cooperation with the Anti-Defamation League of B'Nai B'rith, 1969), p. 4.
4. See Oscar Lewis, *La Vida: A Puerto Rican Family in the Culture of Poverty* (New York: Random House, 1965), pp. xi-xiii.
5. Clarence Senior, *Our Citizens from the Caribbean* (New York: McGraw Hill, 1965), p. 71, and Clarence Senior, *The Puerto Ricans* (Chicago: Quadrangle Books, 1965), p. 38.
6. Richard R. Fagen, Richard A. Brody, and Thomas J. O'Leary, *Cubans in Exile: Disaffection and the Revolution* (Stanford University Press, 1968), pp. 17 ff.
7. For a discussion of some of the problems see *Cuba's Children in Exile: The Story of the Unaccompanied Cuban Refugee Children's Program* (published by the Children's Bureau of the U.S. Department of Health, Education, and Welfare, 1967), and especially the *Cuban Refugee Problem*, a report of the hearings before the Subcommittee to Investigate Problems Connected with Refugees and Escapees, Committee on the Judiciary, United States Senate, in three parts (Washington, D.C.: U.S. Government Printing Office, 1966). See also "Those Amazing Cuban Emigrés," *Fortune*, 74 (October 1966), pp. 144-49.
8. A. Taher Moustafa and Gertrud Weiss, *Health Status and Practices of Mexican Americans*, Mexican-American Study Project, Advance Report II (Los Angeles: University of California, 1968), pp. 5-6.
9. *Ibid.*, pp. 7-11.
10. Martin B. Dworkis, editor, *The Impact of Puerto Rican Migration on Governmental Services in New York City* (New York: New York University Press, 1957), p. 46.
11. *Ibid.*, pp. 46-47.
12. Lawrence R. Chenault, *The Puerto Rican Migrant in New York City* (New York: Columbia University Press, 1938), p. 115.
13. Beatrice Bishop Berle, *Eighty Puerto Rican Families in New York City: Health and Disease Studied in Context* (New York: Columbia University Press, 1958), p. 151.
14. Chenault, *op cit.*, p. 122.
15. Berle, *op. cit.*, p. 122.
16. William Goode, "Illegitimacy in the Caribbean Social Structure," *American Sociological Review*, 25 (February 1960), pp. 21-30.
17. *Ibid.*; and Keith Otterbein, "Caribbean Family," *American Anthropologist*, 67 (1965), pp. 66-79.
18. Berle, *op. cit.*, p. 156.
19. Cervando Martinez and Harry W. Martin, "Folk Diseases Among Urban Mexican-Americans," *Journal of the American Medical Association*, 196 (April 11, 1966), pp. 147-150.

20. Arthur J. Rubel, *Across the Tracks: Mexican Americans in a Texas City* (Austin: University of Texas Press, 1966), pp. 175-193; Lyle Saunders, *Cultural Differences and Medical Care: The Case of the Spanish-Speaking People of the Southwest* (New York: Russell Sage Foundation, 1954), pp. 160-164.
21. Dan Wakefield, *Island in the City: Puerto Ricans in New York* (New York: Corinth Books, 1960), pp. 49-84.
22. Margaret Clark, *Health in the Mexican-American Culture, A Community Study* (Berkeley: University of California Press, 1970), pp. 164-183.
23. George M. Foster, "Relationships Between Spanish and Spanish-American Folk Medicine," *Journal of American Folklore*, 66 (1953), pp. 201-217.
24. Clark, *op. cit.*, pp. 163-217.
25. Saunders, *op. cit.*, p. 147.
26. Martinez and Martin, *op. cit.*, pp. 147-150.
27. Josephine Baca, "Some Health Beliefs of the Spanish Speaking," *American Journal of Nursing*, 69 (October 1969), pp. 2172-2176.
28. See, for example, Oscar Lewis, *The Children of Sanchez* (New York: Vintage Books, 1961).
29. Clark, *op. cit.*, pp. 163-217.
30. Berle, *op. cit.*, p. 159.
31. E. Gartly Jaco, "Mental Health of the Spanish-Americans in Texas," in *Culture and Mental Health*, edited by Marvin Opler (New York: Macmillan, 1959), pp. 467-584.
32. Moustafa and Weiss, *op. cit.*, pp. 31-35.
33. Sam Schulman and Anne M. Smith, "The Concept of Health Among Spanish Speaking Villagers of New Mexico and Colorado," *Journal of Health and Human Behavior,* 4 (Winter 1963), pp. 226-234.

5

The Native Americans

It has been estimated that at least 10,000,000 and perhaps as many as 16,000,000 residents of the United States have some Indian ancestor, or in more technical terms have an ancestor who might be classified as an indigenous native American.[1] These Americans, however, are to be distinguished from the so-called tribal Indians who are the only ones classified as Indians by the United States Census, and who now number approximately 600,000 people. Less than half of the tribal Indians are "pure-blooded" Indians since to the census taker an Indian is a person who resides on a reservation (trust land) or whose name appears on a "tribal roll." Thus an Indian by census definition may be a person with only one-half, one-quarter, one-eighth, or even lesser amounts of Indian ancestry. In fact, during certain periods in our past any Europeans who were married to Indians or to people of mixed bloods were classed as Indians. Today some 410,000 of those classified as Indians live on or near reservations that participate in the programs of the Bureau of Indian Affairs and they furnish the basic subject matter of this chapter.

Interestingly there are large numbers of Indians who are not classed by the United States Government as Indians at all.

Perhaps the largest group are found among the Spanish-speaking Americans, large numbers of whom in Mexico were so classified and who in fact are more or less pure-blooded descendents of the pre-Spanish residents of that country. In Mexico any Indian who moves away from his tribal village and adopts the customs and language of Mexico ceases to be regarded as an Indian, something that large numbers of Indians have done, although great numbers still remain in their native villages. It is also worthy of comment that in the United States large numbers of Indians with Negro ancestors are classed as Negroes by the government even though they have more Indian ancestry than Negro.

Confusion over just who is an Indian is compounded by past policies of the United States Bureau of Indian Affairs which in 1954 admitted that it could not really make an adequate definition of just who an Indian is or was.[2] As a result the term Indian in various government reports can mean a racial grouping, a legal concept, a sociocultural group, or a caste. Today the largest centers of Indian population (as defined by the census) in the United States are Arizona with more than 85,000 Indians; Oklahoma with something more than 65,000; New Mexico with approximately 57,000; Alaska with some 50,000; California and North Carolina, each with about 40,000; South Dakota with some 30,000; and Montana and Washington, each with about 22,000 persons classified as Indians. Tribal lands amount to nearly 40 million acres with an additional 12 million acres in allotted land. Individual reservations range in size from one acre (Strawberry Valley Rancheria in Yuba County, California) to 15 million acres (the Navaho reservation in Arizona, New Mexico, and Utah which is about the size of the state of West Virginia). The eastern states in particular have small communities of Indians like the Pequots in Connecticut, Shinnecocks on Long Island in New York, and the Mattaponys in Virginia who have almost blended into surrounding American society but still maintain their unity and their own cohesive settlements and in some cases enjoy recognition as Indians by the government of the states in which they live.[3]

Prior to the coming of the European settlers to these shores it has been estimated that there were about 600,000 Indians within the forty-eight mainland states, which means that by government count there are now about as many Indians as there were 300 years ago. For a time in the last part of the 19th century it seemed as if the Indian would disappear altogether, and many tribal groupings did, but due in part to a change in government policy the Indian managed to survive and even in some cases, such as the Navaho, to increase. In spite of Hollywood stereotypes the native American Indians were not uniform in physical appearance and their stature and skin tones varied as much as those of the European settlers although all had black hair, brown eyes, and some shade of brown skin. The Winnebagos were noted for their large heads; the Utes for their squat, powerful frames; the Crows for their height. These physical variations, coupled with the hundreds of different dialects belonging to some six major language groups indicate the diversity of the Indian heritage. Culturally they also differed. The Chippewa rode in a birchbark canoe, the Chickasaw in a dugout; the Sac slept in a bark wigwam, the Kiowa in a skin tepee, and the Pueblo in a stone apartment house. The Seminole hunted with a blowgun, the Sioux with a bow. In summary, the American Indians differed as much or more from one another as the English did from the Russians or the French from the Egyptians.

Contact with the oncoming European settlers radically changed the nature of Indian life and although all took something from the new culture some were better able to adjust than others. All, however, came to depend upon the Europeans whether they wanted to or not. The acquisition of metal tools and utensils, firearms, horses, and sheep greatly simplified life for the Indians. Sheep made a new way of life for a few tribes such as the Navaho, but it was the horse which had the greatest impact, and on the plains Indians it created a genuine revolution. The Nez Pearcé, for example, changed from their old subsistence on fishing, root digging, and hunting small animals, to trailing the buffalo herds. The Navahos went so far as to deny their prehorse history by stating that if "there were no horses, there were no Navahos." Some of the Indians such as the Iroquois and the Apaches adopted the European weapons with devastating effect on their Indian neighbors, driving them from choice hunting grounds, seizing their property, and enslaving and killing them. The European penetration forced a wholesale restructuring of Indian political alliances and territorial control, and increasingly the Europeans were the only source for supplies and goods that Indians could not manufacture themselves. Because some of the Indians looked to the French settlers for supplies and others to the British, the wars in Europe had repercussions for the Indians, and the European wars quickly became Indian wars in colonial America. Even if the Indians had all been friendly, which they were not, there would have been Indian wars because of conditions beyond the control of the Indians. Once the United States was founded the Indians continued to fight if only to save their homelands, and all told our forefathers became involved in some 37 Indian wars as they attempted to remove the Indians from the path of their intended settlement.

European settlers also brought diseases with them which sometimes almost annihilated tribes and scattered the panic-stricken survivors. Tuberculosis, syphilis, measles, and smallpox were the principal diseases given to the Indians by the European settlers, although it is possible that syphilis had existed in more quiescent forms before. The Pilgrims regarded it as a sign of divine intervention that some disease, probably smallpox left by visiting sailors, had decimated the Indian population of eastern Massachusetts shortly before their arrival. One of the few tribes whose strength remained unimpaired by the plague, the Pequots, attempted to resist the movement of European settlers into the Connecticut valley in the so-called Pequot War of 1637. During this engagement a small party of whites surrounded the Pequot stronghold during the night, fired it, and killed or burned to death some 500 Indians while losing only two men. Increase Mather, a New England minister, called upon his congregation to thank God for allowing the settlers to send so many "heathen souls to hell." The surviving remnants of the tribe were sold into slavery.[4]

The Pequot War was but a minor skirmish compared to King Philip's War (1675 to 1676) which tended to set the pattern for later American dealings with the Indians. This war, which resulted in nearly 1,000 dead among the settlers, was particularly bitter, and was in part won because so many other Indian groups helped the English settlers. Following the war both hostile and friendly tribesmen alike were required to live in specified villages, were denied arms and ammunition, and were prevented from meeting in assembly. Kept in semiisolation, cut off from their old ways of making a living, the New England Indians entered to rapid decline as they picked up the European vices and diseases faster than they acquired their virtues.

For a time Americans adopted a policy of setting aside certain areas in the West as Indian territory and by 1840 survivors of most of the Eastern tribes had been removed to the West. This practice soon proved a failure largely because Americans themselves continued to move West, coveting the very territory they earlier had granted in perpetuity to the Indians. The great Sioux chief Spotted Tail became so discouraged with the continual government relocation schemes that he rather plaintively asked why the "Great Father" did not "put his red children on wheels, so he can move them as he will?[5]

In the last part of the 19th century there was growing agitation for change in Indian policy as many came to realize that we were in effect exterminating the Indians. One of the most influential forces for change was a woman, Helen Hunt Jackson, a novelist whose *Ramona* was one of the most famous 19th century works of fiction. In 1881 she published *A Century of Dishonor*, an eloquent, impassioned, and biased plea to right the wrongs being done to the Indians and a denunciation of the perfidies of the American government.[6] Part of the difficulty was that the friends of the Indians did not agree on the best way to achieve an equitable solution and yet meet the demands of an expanding America. At first the United States acted as if the Indian nations or tribes were independent foreign powers and made treaties with them. There was growing opposition to regarding Indians as independent subjects, however, and in 1871 Congress stipulated that they were no longer citizens of foreign nations but this did not make them citizens of the United States. The change in the status of the Indians did lead to some benefits; the appropriation of the first sums specifically marked for Indians' education is an example, but at the same time the government made it clear that internal tribal matters could be the subject of national legislation.

Many workers among the Indians felt that the only way Indians could progress was to remove them from the reservation or from the tribal groupings which exercised such dominant influence over them. This kind of recommendation was also favored by groups hostile to the Indians, who coveted the Indian lands and were unable to buy it as long as the tribe itself controlled it. Both groups came together to support the Dawes General Allotment Act of 1887, which was designed to encourage the growth of private enterprise among the Indians. Each adult was to receive

160 acres and each child 80 acres from the tribal lands and the remaining lands were to be sold. Recognizing that most Indians still had no concept of private property, the legislation provided that the allotted lands would be held in trust for 25 years by the government, after which the individual Indian would be granted outright ownership and could sell the land if he wished to do so. The effect upon the Indian was disastrous. As one authority has written, the Dawes Act "may not have civilized the Indian, but it definitely corrupted most of the white men who had any contact with it."[7] Between 1887 and 1934 the Indians lost 86 million of the 138 million acres held by them when the legislation was enacted. Though a small minority of Indians did well by the Dawes Act, and there were several "oil Indians" who made great money through their control of land, for every Indian whose allotment proved to contain oil, there were a score who were reduced to charity. In retrospect, the Dawes Act was extremely unwise and failed to take into account reality; most Indians traditionally had been hunters and gatherers and could not or would not be transformed into farmers overnight. The result was a generation of landless Indians with no vocational training and almost total demoralization.

Only a little more successful was the whole concept behind the development of Indian schools. Again the motivation was rapid assimilation of Indians into the American mainstream although the cupidity so evident in allotting Indians lands was not this time a factor. By 1899 more than $2,500,000 was being expended annually on 148 boarding schools and 225 day schools with almost 20,000 children in attendance. Most of these schools were far removed from the reservation since the educational authorities of the day were in agreement that a complete break with the home environment was essential if the Indians were to become effective citizens. In theory attendance was voluntary, which meant that recruiting students was always a problem. Often the students enrolled at the distant boarding schools were orphans or from families so low in the tribal heirarchy they were unable to resist administrative pressure. Indian parents were generally reluctant to lose their children for months, and death rates among the students were abnormally high. Moreover, many of the skills the Indians were taught in the school had no application to the type of life they would lead when they returned home. This meant that the student who did not adapt to the routine at school was miserable while he was there, but those who did adapt successfully were miserable when they returned home to their families.[8]

The same kind of basic misunderstanding characterized some of the other attempts to force the assimilation of Indians. The Bureau of Indian Affairs for a time ordered reservation officials to slash food and clothing rations on the assumption that this would force the Indians to support themselves. Instead, most of the Indians did what their people traditionally had done—shared what little they had and went hungry together. Officials in Washington also ordered all male Indians to have their hair cut even though some tribesmen believed that long hair had supernatural significance. On at least one reservation refractory Indians were shackled so that the hair cutting could be carried out.

Reasons for the continual misunderstanding of Indian psychology are difficult to come by. It might be that Americans regarded Indians with considerable hostility, and though this hostility might have been a cover-up for deeper feelings of guilt over the maltreatment and exploitation of the Indian, it could not help but be reflected in official policies. Adding to this was the popular stereotype of cultural homogeneity of Indians, which meant that policies all too frequently failed to take into consideration the differences in customs that existed between the tribes. Even though the civil servants who worked for the Bureau of Indian Affairs were often well-educated people, with college or even graduate training, they were usually not trained to understand or work in a culture other than their own.[9] Somehow, in spite of the American misunderstanding, the Indians managed to survive but their living conditions never approached that of their European neighbor.

In examining the Indian past it seems as if the hostility to the Indian often increased with proximity, and those most tolerant were those who had little day-to-day contact. This is most evident in the prohibitions against voting. In 1924, as acknowledgement of American gratitude for the Indians who had served in World War I, the Snyder Act finally conferred citizenship upon all Indians who requested it. Two states with large Indian populations, Arizona and New Mexico, refused to allow Indians to vote until finally in 1948 the Courts ordered them to do so. The Snyder Act, however, seemed to mark an official change in federal governmental attitudes. It was followed two years later by a special study of the Indian under the direction of Lewis Meriam who proposed a sweeping list of reforms including a halt to allotment of land which the report argued had impoverished and demoralized Indians. The full effect of the Meriam recommendations was not felt until the election of Franklin D. Roosevelt, who appointed John Collier as Commissioner of Indian Affairs in 1933.

Collier felt that rather than working for the immediate integration of Indians into American society, the avowed aim of United States policy since 1887, the integrity of the tribe should be supported. He believed in the concept of local community organization and supported tribal leaders even to the point of allocating resources through them rather than to individuals. He, as well as others, argued that the "clan instinct" was dominant among Indians and that tribal operation of assets was a more natural way of administering property than the traditional American concept of private property. He believed that it was only through the tribal system that the Indians could develop self-reliance.[10] The result of his efforts and the recommendations of the Meriam survey was the Wheeler Howard Act of 1934, better known as the Indian Reorganization Act. The Act was an admission that assimilation was still far off although assimilation remained the policy of the United States.

Since the retirement of Collier in 1945 the official policy of the various governmental agencies dealing with Indians has tended to vacillate between one which supports the cultural integrity of the tribal unit and one which encourages integration of Indians into the mainstream of American life. Actually there are problems inherent in both points of view, as evidenced by similar arguments now taking place in Negro communities over black separatism and the preservation of the ghetto culture versus integration. The older policy of encouraging integration sounds reasonable to most Americans but it tended to place a low value on Indian culture and threw the Indian on to the market place ill-equipped to deal with the demands of American life. Traditional Indian values and customs were often treated with disdain by white officials and had low survival values off of the reservation. The result was not only to erect a barrier to effective communication between the Indian and the non-Indian but also in the process to foster feelings of inferiority among the Indians. Assimilation, in effect, proved demoralizing to the vast majority of Indians.

The difficulty with preserving the cultural integrity of the tribal unit, however, is simply that reservation life in the modern American society is an anomaly which makes it difficult to survive. There is no way to earn an adequate living on most reservations. Unemployment rates as high as 33 percent are not uncommon and among some tribes the only employed persons are those who work for a governmental agency or for the tribe itself. Even on those reservations with high employment, underemployment is the norm. Farming on most reservations is at best marginal, if partly because so many reservations were selected by the government because of their poor soil and lack of water. At the present time it is estimated that less than 7 percent of all Indian-held land is suitable for farming.[11] Yet reservations are much too crowded to sustain a hunting or food-gathering economy. Under the tribal policy the individual who decides to leave the reservation must face the fact that Government's policy is to support the tribal unit instead of the individual. This means that he must not only leave behind family and friends, he also has to leave behind his share of community-owned property. Moreover, the various governmental assistant programs for Indians, including health services, are available only to reservation residents. Since the tribal way of life among most of the Indian cultures is a communal one that stresses cooperation rather than competition, the nonreservation Indian is also faced with a whole set of capitalistic norms which tends to make his move from the reservation even more traumatic.

Health and Health Services

Nowhere are the difficulties of American policy toward the Indians more evident than in the delivery of health services. Although Americans tended to discourage and denigrate the Indian medicine man and herbalist, they were usually the only "medical professionals" available until this century. Occasionally civilian or military physicians visited reservations to give medical care but it was not until 1908 that the Bureau of Indian Affairs appointed the first Chief Medical Supervisor. More effective concern was demonstrated in 1910 when Congress appropriated funds to combat the spread of trachoma, an infectious granular conjunctivitis which causes eye damage and even blindness when it is allowed to progress to a chronic state. Trachoma is rarely seen among affluent populations, although it is still endemic in large parts of the Near East and Orient as well as in other areas where poverty and lack of facilities for personal hygiene exist. A survey of Indians made after Congress appropriated the money disclosed that 23 percent of the reservation population had trachoma, with the highest incidence among Oklahoma Indians among whom 69 percent of the people examined had symptoms of the disease. Also showing a high rate of infection were the children in the off-reservation boarding schools,[12] another sign of the difficulties inherent in American policies toward the Indians. Trachoma remained a serious health problem among Indians until the advent of the sulfonamides, but even then its eradication was slowed by the lack of adequate health care. Today the disease is regarded as under control on the reservations, although the residual eye damage left by the earlier ravages of the disease is still reflected in the high rates of blindness among the Indian population.

The findings of trachoma among Indians proved shocking to authorities, and adding further fuel to demand for a change was a survey by the Marine Hospital Health Service in 1913, which revealed the appalling health conditions under which American Indians lived and pointed out that they were lacking in what was regarded as even minimal types of medical care.[13] Making findings and acting effectively to deal with them are, however, two different things. Change came only gradually. In 1924 a Health Division was created within the Bureau of Indian Affairs, and in that same year Public Health nurses were hired. By 1939, however, there were still only 110 Public Health nurses in the service. Dental services had been inaugurated in 1913 but by 1925 there were only seven traveling dentists to cover all the reservations. District medical officers were appointed in 1926 and officers of the Public Health Service Commissioned Corps were detailed to the Indian Bureau, but never in very large numbers. The investigation of Indian affairs commenced by Lewis Meriam in 1926 found Indian health conditions little improved over what they had been in the 1913 report.[14] Many of those active in the Health Service felt that the best solution was to transfer the health program to the Public

Health Service. Agitation for such a transfer had begun as early as 1919 but this was not finally accomplished until the enactment legislation was passed in 1954. Actual transfer took place in 1955 and this has proven to be an extremely important step in upgrading health services. As part of the transfer program the Public Health Service made a comprehensive survey of Indian health problems. The report stated that though the government had long been interested in health services for Indians,

> the American Indian is still the victim of an appalling amount of sickness. The health facilities are either non-existent in some areas, or for the most part obsolescent and in need of repair; personnel housing is lacking or inadequate; workloads have been such as to test the patience and endurance of professional staff. This all points to a gross lack of resources equal to the present load of sickness and accumulated neglect.[15]

One of the groups most deficient in health services in 1955 was the Alaskan natives, a category which included not only the Indians of the southern coastal regions and the interior but the Eskimos farther north and the Aleuts who lived in the Aleutian islands as well as on the coast of Alaska. Neither of these last two groups are Indians but the problem of the Alaskan natives emphasizes the problems which the Indians had. Though the vast distances in Alaska, as well as the hostile climate impose great difficulties, the report pointed out that in 1954 there were 600 beds available for patients in the six hospitals which admitted natives even though there were 2,452 new tuberculosis cases reported in that year in addition to all other types of illness requiring hospitalization.[16]

With the incorporation of Indian health services into the Public Health Service, appropriations for Indian medical care expanded rapidly. Observers of the Congressional scene, as well as the supporters of the transfer, believe that a major reason for the increase in funds is that Congress no longer has to appropriate money specifically for Indian health services, an act which apparently still had considerable political opposition, but instead they could appropriate it for general public health and the section on Indian health did not receive the same hostile scrutiny and publicity that a separate appropriation would. Whatever the cause, the appropriations rose from $35 million in 1956,[17] to $109 million in 1969.[18] At present the Indian Health Service operates some 51 hospitals, 77 health centers, and more than 300 health stations and field clinics. It also contracts with various state and community facilities for care because reservations are still so scattered and population so dispersed that public health facilities are not always within reach. Coverage is available to approximately 410,000 individuals[19] on some 250 reservations or native villages (as is the case of Alaskan natives). Excluded from the program are all Indians who have left the reservation as well as Indians in California and elsewhere who live on reservations but whose health care by agreement with the Indians and with the state is under the jurisdiction of state and local health departments.[20]

As a result of these developments in Indian health care, the improvements in Indian health within the last few years have been remarkable. However, even the best health care delivery system cannot fully overcome the effects of poverty and malnutrition and the stress of rapid social change. Life expectancy for Indians in 1965 was estimated at 63.5, which means that their death rate was as high or higher than that of any other minority ethnic group.[21] The infant mortality rate, which fell from 62.5 per 1,000 in 1955 to 32.2 by 1967, was still at that time 1.4 times the national average.[22] Table 1 shows a comparison of the causes of death for Indians and Alaskan natives compared with the overall rates for the general population. Significant differences are evident in the nature and types of the causes of death and show some of the difficulties still facing the Indians. Fatal accidents, for example, are more than three times as common among Indians as among the rest of the population and are the leading cause of death. Further investigation into the accident rate shows that between the ages of 25 and 45 the fatalities are five times that of the comparable population and that this rate has increased since 1955 while other types of death have declined.[23] The accident statistics in part reflect such factors as unsafe vehicles, poor housing, and unsafe working conditions, but they also indicate a much more serious problem. Further evidence of this problem is faced by looking at the suicide rate, which is nearly twice the national average; the homicide rate, which is three times the national average; and deaths from cirrhosis of the liver, which are more than four times as common among Indians as among other Americans.[24] It seems

TABLE 1. Cause of Death for Indians and Alaskan Natives Compared with the Cause of Death for Americans in General (Calendar Year 1967)

Cause of Death	Indian and Alaskan Natives		Total Population	
	No.	%	No.	%
All causes	4,776	100.0	1,851,323	100.0
Accidents	1,000	20.9	113,169	6.1
Diseases of the heart	774	16.2	721,268	39.0
Malignant neoplasms	392	8.2	310,983	16.8
Influenza and pneumonia*	296	6.2	56,892	3.1
Diseases of early infancy	273	5.7	48,314	2.6
CNS vascular lesions	270	5.7	202,184	10.9
Cirrhosis of the liver	215	4.5	27,816	1.5
Homicide	110	2.3	13,425	0.7
Diabetes mellitus	107	2.2	35,049	1.9
Suicide	94	2.0	21,325	1.2
Tuberculosis	90	1.9	6,901	0.4
Gastritis, etc.	80	1.7	7,504	0.4
All other causes	1,075	22.5	286,493	15.5

*Excludes the newborn.

Source: Indian Health Service, Trends and Services, 1969 Edition, U.S. Department of Health, Education, and Welfare (Washington, D.C.: U.S. Government Printing Office, 1969), p. 16.

evident that many of the deaths not labeled as suicide seem to be self-destructive in nature and to suggest that Indians are facing almost insolvable social problems.

The situation which has been created for them is not unlike the conditions of anomie described by the French sociologist, Emile Durkheim. Though Durkheim made his generalizations on the basis of rapid social changes created by industrialization, they would seem to apply to any society undergoing rapid social change which causes old norms to lose their saliency without their being immediately replaced with new rules which are functional. Durkheim said that during this period of adjustment people are unsure of themselves or torn between conflicting sets of norms so that social pathology such as suicide is common.[25]

The extent of the anomie caused by the conflicting life styles varies among the tribes. Many Indians, including most of those who still live east of the Mississippi River, had already accepted European customs before the advent of the reservation era so that their time of great trauma was behind them. In some of the western tribes the problem of transition is acute. Some individuals, particularly the older Indians, are still well adjusted to the old traditions, but others, particularly young adults, are caught in an identity crisis and are unable to find a satisfactory life-style either as traditionally oriented Indians or as members of the mainstream of American society.[26] If they stay on the reservation, they are caught in a crippling web of poverty, unemployment, and dependency on welfare. If they leave the reservation to find employment, the jobs which are available are often seasonal, low-paying, or hazardous, and in the case of forest-fire fighting, which the western tribesmen perform, it is all three. The feelings of ambivalence and hopelessness that follow from this seemingly impossible situation are expressed in various other ways besides suicide. Although most Indian children now get some education, the drop-out rate is so high that few Indians achieve the level of education necessary for skilled employment in today's world.[27]

Alcoholism traditionally has been a severe problem among Indians and for long periods in American history it was forbidden to sell alcohol to Indians. The 1953 repeal of this prohibition was an important reform in that it removed one more vestige of white paternalism, but this did not by any means solve the problem.[28] Either because of a carryover from the time when drinking was forbidden and alcohol was consumed rapidly to avoid apprehension, or because alcohol helps drown one's problems, large numbers of Indians still consume liquor so rapidly and in such great quantity that drunkenness inevitably follows. The inebriated Indians are then killed by trains, automobiles, or even by their companions.[29] If they survive their drinking bout they are often thrown into jail where they can easily develop pneumonia, and if they survive this crisis as well, large numbers ultimately die of cirrhosis of the liver.

Another health problem which continues to plague Indians is tuberculosis. In the 1913 health survey it was found that only the relatively assimilated Indian populations of New York and Michigan had low tuberculosis rates. On the western reservations it was not unusual to find 20 percent of a tribe afflicted and among the Paiutes of the Pyramid Lake Region in Nevada some 33 percent had the disease. Since this survey was made before such diagnostic tools as x-ray or the tuberculin tests were available and depended only upon a physical examination, the true incidence may well have been higher than the figures reported.[30] In spite of the advances made in recent years, the mortality rate for tuberculosis is still five times as high for Indians as for the general population. When the age-adjusted rate is used to compensate for the relatively youthful age of the Indian population (because of the lower longevity rates) the tuberculosis rate is eight times as high as that of the general population.[31] Because tuberculosis has been such a serious menace to Indian survival, there were some experts in the early part of the 20th century who believed that Indians had some special genetic susceptibility to the disease. This idea has now been discarded and current research suggests that the high incidence is more closely related to poverty and inadequate living conditions than to any other factor.[32]

Among the Navaho, the largest of the modern Indian tribes, tuberculosis was a major cause of death and suffering until the last few years. It is estimated that in the period following World War II tuberculosis in some form or another affected one out of every ten Navahos. The situation was so bad that mobile case findings and roentgenographic surveys were abandoned because there were not enough facilities available to hospitalize the known cases. When Isoniazid was developed in 1952 the early field trials of the drug were undertaken on the reservation simply because there were so many cases regarded as medically hopeless. Physicians from Cornell University treated 30 cases of miliary tuberculosis, a form considered fatal because infection is rapidly spread throughout the body through the bloodstream. Some 28 of the patients were saved, which meant that if the drug could cure such severe cases it would be even more effective against other forms of tuberculosis.

Elsewhere in this book we have criticized the tendency of the medical establishment to use either poverty-stricken or minority populations as testing grounds to perfect individual skills or try out new therapies which are later used on their middle-class patients. The experimental use of Isoniazid should be differentiated from this type of experimentation since, while the Navahos were the research subjects, they were also among the worst sufferers from the disease and the follow-through treatment was concentrated on the very group which most needed it, the Indians themselves. It is not drug experimentation which should be condemned but the use of subjects who as a group do not receive the major benefits from the experimentation.

With the development of Isoniazid and similar drugs, the technology was available for the control of tuberculosis. The entrance of the Public Health Service into the field after 1955 made the necessary medical services available and within a few years the disease was brought to its present level of control. The fact that tuberculosis still remains such a serious problem seems to emphasize again that adequate medical care cannot solve all the problems, and that low socioeconomic status and cultural and geographic barriers still act as effective deterrents to good health.

Both poverty and geographic barriers also seem to be implicated in the infant mortality rates resulting for the most part from pneumonia or diarrhea. Infant diarrhea can usually be treated successfully if steps are taken soon enough to restore the fluid and electrolyte balance. The physical isolation of many reservation residents and the uncertain condition of their vehicles often cause the family to put off the trip to the hospital until it is too late. Moreover, crowded living quarters and lack of sanitation help communicable diseases to spread, and an inadequate diet predisposes to illness. If the Indian population is to be a healthy one problems associated with poverty and isolation must be solved.

Some effective strides have been taken by the Indian Health Service to overcome some of the cultural and communication barriers to health care which existed earlier. One of the most effective ways has been to hire as many Indians and Alaskan natives as possible,[33] but until recently most such employees were hired at low levels either because of their poor educational preparation or because of the rigidity of the health professions in demanding certain traditional forms of education. In fact, until anthropologists emphasized the importance of the Indian medicine man, medical workers opposed him, which only served to make the Indians more suspicious of the white health worker. Even as recently as 1945 the medicine man among the Navaho had a preferred status over the physician, which meant that if there was a conflict between the two, scientific medicine lost out. Among the Pueblo Indians the councils often still retain control over day-to-day actions to the extent that permission must be granted by the Council before a mother can allow a public health official to inoculate a child. Recognition of the importance of Indian customs by the modern health workers has tended to cut down some of the hostility between the Indian and Western medicine, and this hostility has further decreased as more effective attempts have been made to use Indians in more creative ways as health educators, home health aides, and other types of health workers. Presently the roles of physician's assistant and nurse practitioner are being considered and a few tentative steps have been taken, but there is no large-scale program to train Indian professionals in these roles. It would seem that at least on the western reservations the great distances and the isolation of the people would tend to encourage the growth of such workers. If the Indian is to care for himself such workers would also be a necessity since in the past medical schools have tended to bar Indians from admission and this means that even as medical schools begin to change there will still be a shortage of indigenous physicians for a long time.

It is particularly important that indigenous workers be developed now that the Indian view of Western medicine has become so much more favorable. Among the Navaho, for example, the crucial factor in changing long-term suspicion into favorable support has been the success in the treatment of tuberculosis by Western medicine. Until this happened all Western medicine was able to do was offer palliative therapy, which was not too different or any more effective than what the medicine man could offer; besides, the medicine man kept the person at home instead of sending him off to the hospital to die. In fact, Western medicine found itself in a circuitous web. Indians often turned to Western medicine only when the medicine man had given up on treatment, and then the sick Indian was taken off to a hospital where he did indeed die. It was only when the Indian could see that the Western medicine was actually doing some good that he began to believe that it had some merit. Now, although the medicine man is still important among many tribal groups for ceremonial healing rites, he is considered an alternative or religious approach to healing that does not preclude the use of Western therapy.[34]

Though the Indian health seems to be getting better today, it is still too early to indicate that the problems are really under control. Much of the recent advance has been due to the fact that young physicians took the Indian Health Service as an alternative to the Armed Forces in the medical draft. This tended to increase the number of physicians available, although many of them lacked the necessary skills really to accomplish what was needed. As draft calls recede the numbers of available physicians will also recede and this means that the Public Health Service will need to launch more intensive recruitments. Even if they are successful and have the funds to carry through, there will be difficulty because the Indians are so widely dispersed—at least in the western states—that a physician who works among the Indians is able to accomplish much less than he would in a more concentrated urban center. This again emphasizes the need for more indigenous paramedical personnel.

Decreases in Indian mortality figures are also dependent upon decreasing malnutrition, improving sanitation, and raising the level of employment. Health care in itself is not enough. Obviously the Indians of today are much better off than they were just a few years ago, at least as far as general health standards are concerned, but they still have a long way to go to meet the standards of the more affluent Americans. Cultural conflict is still a problem, and the anomie and feelings of hopelessness created by this conflict are still evident. In the long run the only effective way to overcome the remaining health problems is to deal with base causes, starting with the problem of poverty.

Notes

1. Jack D. Forbes, editor, *The Indian in America's Past* (Englewood Cliffs, N.J.: Prentice Hall, 1964), pp. 3-4.
2. See the testimony of Leonard M. Hill, Sacramento Area Director, Bureau of Indian Affairs, as reported in the *Progress Report to the Legislature by the Senate Interim Committee on Indian Affairs* (Sacramento: California State Senate, 1955), pp. 241-242, 407-408.
3. Alvin M. Josephy, Jr., *The Indian Heritage of America* (New York: Alfred A. Knopf, 1969), pp. 359-60.
4. William T. Hagan, *American Indians* (Chicago: University of Chicago, 1961), p. 13.
5. *Ibid.*, p. 121.
6. See Helen Maria Hunt Jackson, *A Century of Dishonor,* new edition edited by Andrew F. Rolle (reprinted, New York: Harper & Row, 1965).
7. Hagan, *op. cit.*, p. 146.
8. *Ibid.*, pp. 134-135.
9. Harold E. Fey and D'Arcy McNickle, *Indians and Other Americans: Two Ways of Life* (New York: Harper & Brothers, 1959), p. 195.
10. Hagan, *op. cit.*, p. 156.
11. *Health Service for American Indians*, prepared by the Office of Surgeon General, U.S. Department of Health, Education, and Welfare, Public Health Service Publication No. 531 (Washington, D.C.: U.S. Government Printing Office, 1957), p. 28.
12. *Ibid.*, Appendix C, pp. 261-262.
13. Bertram S. Kraus, *Indian Health in Arizona* (Tucson: University of Arizona Press, 1954), p. 4.
14. For a summary of the report see *Health Service for American Indians*, Appendix C, Report II, pp. 264-269.
15. *Ibid.*, p. vii.
16. Division of Indian Health, Program Analysis and Special Studies Branch, *Eskimos, Indians and Aleuts of Alaska*, part of U.S. Department of Health, Education, and Welfare Report on *Indians on Federal Reservations* (Washington, D.C.: U.S. Government Printing Office, 1963), pp. 7-8.
17. *Health Service for American Indians*, p. 98.
18. Indian Health Service, *To the First Americans: The Third Annual Report on the Indian Health Program of the U.S. Public Health Service* (Washington, D.C.: U.S. Government Printing Office, 1969), p. 13.
19. U.S. Department of Health, Education, and Welfare, *Nursing Careers Among the American Indians*, Public Health Service, 1970, p. 1.
20. U.S. Division of Indian Health, *Indians on Federal Reservation in the United States, Phoenix Area: Arizona, California, Nevada, Utah*, U.S. Department of Health, Education, and Welfare, Public Health Service Publication No. 615, Part 6 (January 1961), p. 32.
21. Senator and Mrs. Fred R. Harris, "Indian Health," in *Sources: A Blue Cross Report of Health Problems of the Poor* (Chicago: Blue Cross Association, 1968), pp. 38-43.

22. Indian Health Services, *Trends and Services, 1969 Edition*, U.S. Department of Health, Education, and Welfare (Washington, D.C.: U.S. Government Printing Office, 1969), p. 8.
23. *Ibid.*, p. 25.
24. *Ibid., passim*, and also Indian Health Service, *Suicide Among the American Indians*, U.S. Public Health Service Publication No. 1903 (Washington, D.C.: U.S. Government Printing Office, 1967).
25. Emile Durkheim, *Suicide: A Study in Sociology*, translated from the French by John A. Spaulding and George Simpson (Glencoe, Ill.: The Free Press, 1951).
26. Roy Bongarts, "Who Am I? The Indian Sickness," *The Nation*, (April 27, 1970), pp. 496-498.
27. Harris, *op. cit.*
28. John Adair and Kurt W. Deuschle, *The People's Health: Medicine and Anthropology in a Navaho Community* (New York: Appleton-Century-Crofts, 1970), and Harris, *op. cit.*
29. Personal communication from Pamela Brink, based upon her studies of Paiute Reservation life.
30. *Health Service for American Indians*, Appendix C, p. 262.
31. *Trends and Services, 1969 Edition*, pp. 16-18.
32. J. G. Townsend, "Indian Health—Past, Present, and Future," in *The Changing Indian*, edited by Oliver LaFarge (Norman: University of Oklahoma Press, 1942), pp. 28-41.
33. *Ibid.*
34. John Adair and Kurt W. Deuschle, *op. cit.*, pp. 1-13, 21.

6

Poverty and Hunger Transcend Racial Lines

There is a widespread general assumption among Americans that only members of minority groups are likely to be poor. Many people, even those from poverty backgrounds, do not seem to realize the extent of poverty in the United States or its implications for the health of the nation. The president of a local chapter of the National Association for the Advancement of Colored People, a sincere and thoughtful man, stated in a recent speech:

> *I really do not understand how a white person can be poor. In the town I grew up in the whites had everything. They went to the brick school and they owned all of the stores. They lived in the best houses and had all the advantages. It seems impossible that a white person would be poor unless he is lazy or stupid.*

For this reason, if for no other, it seems essential to state that in 20th century America, it is still possible to be white and poor without being lazy or stupid. Poverty transcends racial lines.

White poverty exists for many of the same reasons that poverty exists among the various nonwhite minority groups: insufficient education, lack of employment opportunities or chances for advancement, too many children, poor geographic location, age, and the cycle of poverty itself, which creates feelings of powerlessness and hopelessness that make success difficult. Many people whose income was once adequate can fall below the poverty line in their later years because social security or old age assistance programs do not provide incomes which are comparable to the income levels of most people before retirement. Even those individuals who were able to save or invest some of their income during their more productive years run into difficulty because inflation has devalued their possessions and investments. Moreover, there are some aged persons who, though very much in need of assistance, are given no welfare aid. Some of these people through ignorance have never applied and welfare departments do not usually seek out possible recipients. Others have attempted to get some assistance but were turned down because they cannot prove their age or because they encounter some other technicality. Because of these various factors, in 1966 two out of five households defined as consisting of one aged person or an elderly couple fell below the poverty line, as compared with one in seven in other households.[1]

Others who fall into the poverty classification are victims of technological changes which have made their occupational skills worthless. The largest and most significant group to which this last category applies makes its living from farm-related occupations. Presently there are 14,000,000 rural Americans who fall below the poverty line. They constitute 40 percent of the nation's poor although only 30 percent of the total population is rural. The overwhelming bulk of the rural poor—eleven of the fourteen million—are white, which means that while the urban poor compose a mosaic of ethnic identities, the rural poor are predominantly poor white from old American stock.[2]

In the revolutionary age of the 20th century, one of the most revolutionary changes in many ways has been in the nature of agriculture. The extent of the agricultural revolution is indicated from the fact that in 1822 it took some 50 to 60 man hours to raise 20 bushels of wheat; by 1890 this had dropped to 8 or 10 hours, and by 1930 to 3 or 4 hours. The rate has since continued to drop so that both in percentages and in absolute numbers it takes fewer people to raise more than ever before. In the United States some 18.7 percent of the total population was actively engaged in agriculture in 1940; by 1950 the percentage had dropped to 12.2; by 1960, to 7.8; by 1965, to 5.9; and today it is around 5 percent. In the process the basic farm unit has changed from the small farmer, or tenant farmer, to a big business with specialized money crops, and those farmers who have survived have tremendous sums of money invested in equipment, land, and know-how.

While in the long run revolutions are often beneficial, they are usually brought about with tremendous human suffering. The agricultural revolution is no exception to this general rule, and though many people have left farming voluntarily, particularly those of the younger generation, many others have been forced off the land by depression, lack of investment capital, and inability to make a living. Moreover, many still live on farms which economically are no longer feasible although they scratch out a living. Within the past half century the small American farmer has led a precarious existence. World War I led to an artificial inflation in farm prices, and farmers expanded and bought equipment to take advantage of it. The farm price index reached a high of 211 in 1920 but it fell to 121 in 1921, and though it rose slightly thereafter, it fell to a new low of 68 in 1932. The result was forced sales due to bankruptcies, foreclosures, and tax delinquencies, which increased from an average of 12 per 1,000 farms in 1921 to 54 per 1,000 in 1933. Since many of the people who had lost their farms were unskilled, as were the farm laborers who were also forced onto the market, they sought the lowest-paying jobs in the cities or migrated elsewhere to find farm work. Large numbers of residents of Texas, Oklahoma, and Arkansas, whose economic plight was worsened by the "dust bowl" of the period, migrated to California in search of jobs in the fruit and vegetable fields. As we mentioned in an earlier chapter, John Steinbeck's *The Grapes of Wrath* painted a classic picture of this displaced group as it slowly worked its way westward. Today, more than half of the people born in such states as Arkansas no longer live there.

The average size of farms of all kinds increased from about 150 acres in the 1930s to over 300 acres in the 1960s, mostly through the elimination of small farms. In fact, an estimated 2,500,000 farms were eliminated during the 30-year period and an equal number of farm families displaced. Large numbers of farms today are still economically not paying their way, and the elimination continues. Increasingly the farmer has either to expand radically to justify his investment in equipment or sell out to still larger owners. Some still hang on, trying to supplement their farm wages with a job in the nearby town, but such jobs are increasingly difficult to obtain as the small town itself is hit by the changing nature of agriculture. Small town merchants, businessmen, tradesmen, and others have perhaps undergone as radical a change as the farmer as America becomes increasingly urbanized. The extent of their dilemma is evidenced from the fact that only one-fourth of the rural poor actually live on farms; the other three-fourths of them live in the small towns and villages. Job opportunities in the rural towns are scarce and becoming scarcer, and eventually many of these people will be forced to migrate to major urban centers without the grub stake that the sale of farm land might have given them. Unfortunately large numbers of the rural poor are handicapped in seeking jobs when they do move to the city because of their low educational level, which averages only about 8.8 years of schooling.[3]

Still another factor which has handicapped the farmer in his struggle against poverty is the size of his family. Though it is a truism that high birth rates tend to correlate with low educational and income levels, there is also a cultural lag involved as far as rural Americans are concerned. This is because before the era of the mechanized farm a large family was an economic asset since so many hands were needed to carry out the work on the farm. Although the trend is downward, rural families are still somewhat larger than urban ones.[4]

Rural poverty exists everywhere in the United States but there are groups of people who face a more desperate situation than others, such as the residents of the southern Appalachians, most of whom are white, the southern farmers outside of Appalachia, many of whom are black, and the migrant farm workers throughout the country, who tend to have mixed ethnic identities. Although Mexican-American farm laborers are predominant in the western states, in other areas of the country this is not the case.

Appalachia

One of the most troubled regions in terms of economic difficulties, and which can serve as a mirror for other areas, is the southern Appalachians—variously defined, but which include parts of Alabama, Georgia, Tennessee, North Carolina, Virginia, Kentucky, and West Virginia. Some surveys also include parts of Maryland or South Carolina, which are on the fringe of the area. The hard core, however, covers 190 counties, is some 600 miles long, and nearly 250 miles across at its widest point. It encompasses approximately 80,000 square miles, and in the 1960 census contained 5,672,178 people. The region was identified as a problem area first in the 1930s when the United States Department of Agriculture concluded that the area held the highest concentration of low-income farms in the country; moreover, the density of farm population was much greater than in the richest agricultural areas of the Middle West but without any real major cash crop. The Cumberland Plateau area, included in the Appalachian area, stood out as the lowest income group in United States agriculture in the middle 1930s, with a gross income per farm inhabitant of less than $150 in most of the counties. Six counties had more than half their population on relief during the depression. A study made in the 1930s concluded that 350,000 people should leave the region's agriculture, and that 60,000 should leave mining—this *before* the current radical changes in farming. In this region, the depression, through its public programs, actually raised living standards for many families who previously had lacked contact with the American standard of living. The region remained one with a high rate of relief and a low basis for economic security. Self-employment and a deficit of large-scale industry left many occupations uncovered by social security, thus placing a double burden on welfare agencies. In addition, residential requirements for aid, which have only recently been modified, served to immobilize many workers and their families in problem areas.[5]

Although Appalachia is now becoming less isolated than it once was, and more industrialized, parts of the area still lag behind the rest of the nation. The small Appalachian farmers, perhaps the last of the "rugged individualists," live on subsistence farms which grow only a few staples, so they cannot afford to cut back production to benefit from the federal government's crop subsidies program. They need to plant all of their land in order to have enough yield to feed their families, yet the overuse of the soil has in the long run decreased that production, so their situation is a deteriorating one. The small coal mining enterprises also continue to fail, as other types of fuel replace coal, and in many areas there is no other alternative employment. Because of this depressed economic situation Appalachians receive more outside relief from government, church, and private agencies in proportion to their contribution than any other area of comparable size in the nation.[6] The very factors which once had survival value in the region—a dogged independence, a suspicion of outsiders, and a low value for education—today serve to perpetuate the poverty of the area, and when Appalachians migrate to cities outside of the areas these qualities act as barriers to their success and acceptance in the urban environment.[7]

Still migration seems to be one way of solving the area's problems and during the 10 years between 1950 and 1960 the Southern Appalachia Region lost more than one million persons, a number equal to a fifth of the total population in 1950. As a result the 1960 census revealed a regional population decrease for the first time since the region was settled.[8] Since the migrant population was made up primarily of young adults between 18 and 34 years of age, the number of persons in dependent ages, particularly those under 15 and over 65, rose in the area. This further complicated the problems of those who have stayed because it was the most vigorous people who had left.

Many of the migrants have gone to cities in the South such as Atlanta or Birmingham, but those in the northern part of the area flow northward into Baltimore, Washington, Cincinnati, Cleveland, Chicago, Dayton, Detroit, and other major cities. Although Appalachians are of old American stock and could popularly be termed WASPs (white, Anglo-Saxon Protestants*), in the large northern urban areas they are treated as a minority group. There are Appalachian enclaves in the slums that border the black and Puerto Rican settlements and replace the Italians and Poles who are moving to the suburbs. The talk and the folk wisdom is from "down home" rather than from a foreign country, but the poverty, the underemployment, the big families, the inadequate housing, and the discouragement is the same as it is in the parts of the slums in which members of ethnic minority groups live.

Migrant Farm Workers

More widely dispersed is another form of rural poverty, namely, that of the farm wage worker, many of whom are migrant workers. As the number and nature of farms have declined, so has the number of hired workers. In 1950 a total of 2,329,000 were working for pay during the survey week selected by the Department of Agriculture. In 1969 the number had dropped to 1,174,000 (more than 50 percent). Most of the paid workers were nonmigratory workers who lived in the community and supplemented their income during rush times in the agricultural cycle. Large numbers of them, however, were migratory workers, and in 1968 there were still about 300,000 so classified.[9] Average daily salary for the migratory workers was $11.15 in 1968 for those 20 years of age or older, and $8.15 for those 19 or under.

There are three major streams of migratory workers. One group spends the winter in Florida and Georgia, harvesting winter crops and moving northward through the Atlantic states in the summer and returning late in the fall; a second group moves northward from Texas and spreads out through the Central states, while a third stream is centered in California and the Pacific states. As the workers usually travel as a family or in small groups, there are large variations in case histories of individuals and families.

*Actually most Appalachians are descendents of Scotch-Irish ancestors, so they are not technically "Anglo-Saxons," but the term WASP has an elastic interpretation. Appalachians are clearly white and Protestant.

They indicate quite different patterns prompted by hope, rumor, and sometimes even accurate job information or contracts. Though many of the migrant workers are members of ethnic minority groups, large numbers are white.

Some casual observers of the migrant workers have claimed that farm migrancy exists because of the seasonal labor requirements of agriculture and that the people become migrants because they like the life. Neither of these generalizations seems valid on investigation in most cases, although a few crops do demand intense attention for only one or two weeks. Investigators have found that the majority of American-born migrant farm workers seem to be victims of either occupational displacement, racial discrimination, illiteracy, or poor health, or accidents, and they have turned to farm labor to survive. In effect, seasonal farm work in the past has provided an opportunity for those who are not qualified for or are not accepted in the more desirable occupations.

Migratory farm workers, although on the lowest rung of the economic ladder and the most in need, were excluded from the protection of major national and state statutes dealing with working and living conditions until the last few years. They were not covered by unemployment insurance, had no right to organize, lacked protection of minimum wage guarantees, and had little say about their working conditions. They also had little political power because few were able to meet the residence requirements for voting, and the lack of guarantee for them to organize meant that they lacked the protection group efforts might have given them. Their economic difficulties are complicated by the fact that they travel as a family unit, and this means that their children also suffer. To eke out a living everyone who is able to work, including children, go to the fields, although many states now prevent those under 14 from working. Little supervision is given to the children while the mother is in the field and the accident rate among these children is high. Schooling for children of migratory workers is inadequate because long periods are spent on the road and distances between jobs are great. Housing is mainly improvised, and medical care in the past has been most non-existent. Education, child care, health and sanitation are difficult enough under migratory conditions, but when this is compounded by the uncertainty of employment and by real poverty the results are too often deplorable.

Health Problems of the Poor

Most of the health problems associated with poverty have been mentioned before because they are the same kind of problems faced by minority group members, most of whom are also poor. Whatever their ethnic identity the members of the poverty population are much more likely to die of contagious diseases than the general population, and because they die younger they are less likely to die of malignant neoplasms and cardio-vascular diseases. Maternal and infant mortality rates, naturally, are higher for the poverty group. Poverty itself is not listed on the death certificate because poverty is not an illness; instead, it has to be classed as a major contributing factor in many deaths. Some of the reasons are obvious. With our present health care system a lack of funds acts as a barrier to adequate medical care, which means that untreated or improperly treated illness is more common among the poor and that major health crises are more likely to occur. Overcrowded living conditions and lack of sanitary facilities are major contributors to the spread of infectious diseases. One aspect of poverty and health that has not been so widely publicized, however, is the correlation between poverty and malnutrition.

Using the Social Security Administration index, $3,743 was set as a minimum amount adequate to feed, clothe, and house a non-farm family of four in 1969. Smaller families had a corresponding reduction in their estimated essential income and larger families a corresponding increase. By these standards, some 24.3 million persons or about one tenth of the nation's families were classified as poor. If the calculations of the Social Security Administration were correct, and this was in fact an essential minimum, then the conclusion becomes obvious: these families, including large numbers on welfare, do not feed, clothe, or house themselves or their children adequately. Since rent tends to be a fixed expense, it is often met first, and the problem then becomes that of feeding the family until the next check arrives. This means that many people have periods of going without a meal. The extent of this hunger was revealed in a California survey which disclosed that 44 percent of the children on AFDC (Aid to

Families with Dependent Children) in Sacramento County had involuntarily gone without food one or more days during the year because the family had run out of money to buy food.[11]

Hunger is by no means a new phenomenon in America or elsewhere, although much of the public concern over malnutrition is of fairly recent origin. In the winter of 1965-1966, 35 Negroes invaded an abandoned air force base in Greenville, Mississippi, because they said they were hungry, cold, and unemployed. Federal troops were sent in to evict the demonstrators but a federal interdepartmental committee was set up to investigate the claims of the 35 that they and other residents of the area were starving.[12] Eventually, a delegation of United States Senators visited Mississippi in April 1967 to investigate poverty and hunger. The committee was shocked by what they saw. One member of the delegation, Senator George Murphy of California, regarded as one of the more conservative members, indicated that he was unprepared for what he saw. "I didn't know that we were going to be dealing with the situation of starving people and starving youngsters."[13]

The chairman of the investigating committee, Joseph S. Clark of Pennsylvania, briefly summarized the findings:

> We saw families who, without income with which to buy food or food stamps, were suffering from the effects of acute malnutrition and hunger. It is an exercise in semantics to argue whether these and other families about whom we have heard and of whom we will hear today are "starving." Senator [Robert] Kennedy of New York observed that the conditions he saw in the delta were as bad as any he had seen in his extensive tour of South America. One of the doctors who will testify today, and who has had extensive experience in Africa has said that conditions he observed in this country are as bad or worse than those in Kenya and Aden.[14]

Testifying before the committee was a panel of six physicians who, with financial support from the Field Foundation, had made a personal inspection of the conditions in Mississippi with respect to malnutrition and medical care. These men reported that school children were unable to learn because of hunger and that signs of malnutrition were widespread. One of them reported that in an examination of a sample of 501 preschool children, it was found that 81 percent of them were anemic, with hemocrit readings below 35. The diet of many Mississippi children was found to be practically devoid of animal protein. To complicate matters, the group reported that there was widespread evidence of discrimination in health care. One member went on to state a widespread belief that there was an unwritten but generally accepted policy on the part of those who controlled the state to try to drive Negroes out of the state or eliminate them by starving them to death.[15]

As might be expected, the report of these physicians to the Senate and to the world caused an uproar. Mississippi Senators James O. Eastland and John Stennis objected to the findings of both the Field Foundation project and the Senate subcommittee. They produced witnesses who argued that the reports were biased and unfair, and that Mississippi had wrongfully been singled out because hunger existed elsewhere.[16] On this last point the two Mississippi senators had the facts on their side. The Office of Economic Opportunity reported that hunger was a problem not only in Mississippi but also among Alaskan natives, the urban poor, rural Appalachia, and elsewhere.[17] The focus of the investigation of the problem of hunger widened from what had seemed to be a Mississippi tragedy to a national problem, and the Senate committee went on to hold hearings and hear witnesses from throughout the country.

In the summer of 1967 a Citizens Crusade Against Poverty was set up with Benjamin E. Mays, President Emeritus of Morehouse College in Atlanta, and Leslie Dunbar, Executive Director of the Field Foundation, as co-chairmen. This group also held hearings and collected data about the problems of hunger. Their findings were in substantial agreement with the findings of the official Senate subcommittee and other investigations carried out by journalists. Hunger, it was suddenly agreed, was a widespread phenomenon in this country and the consequences of chronic malnutrition were found to be serious and widespread.

The incidence of anemia among poor infants was found to be particularly high. In a Washington, D.C. study of 460 children from low-income families, 29 percent were found to be anemic, with the highest rate recorded between the ages of 12 and 17 months, when 65 percent were so classified.[18] Similar statistics were found to be true for Chicago, New York, Pittsburgh, and Baltimore.[19] In the Senate hearings physicians testified that the anemia they saw in small children tended to complicate other illnesses. One Kentucky pediatrician reported that the children from poor families spent twice as long in the hospital as those from more well-to-do families because the handicaps of parasites and malnutrition tended to slow their recovery rate.[20]

Though there were few large-scale or carefully controlled research projects reported in these hearings on hunger, the cumulative evidence of reports by physicians who had examined the poverty population or who had compared patients across income levels was overwhelming. Large numbers of poor children not only did not have adequate diets, many were actually hungry. One of the ways this poor diet showed up clinically was in the development of nutritional anemia, a result of either iron or protein deficiencies. This anemia was most often manifest in infants below the age of two, in part because they are unable to eat the regular family diet, but also because their nutritional needs are so great during this most rapid growth period.

Investigators found even more serious protein deficiencies among some of the American Indians,[21] so serious that they were diagnosed as having kwashiorkor and marasmus, conditions usually associated with the most economically deprived areas of the world. Earlier research had also reported kwashiorkor among the children of migrant farm workers in Florida.[22] Marasmus is the term applied to a generalized undernutrition in which the intake of protein, calories, vitamins, and iron are all inadequate. Kwashiorkor is an old African tribal name for the syndrome which was frequently observed when infants were displaced from the breast by the birth of a younger sibling. The outstanding clinical symptom of kwashiorkor which differentiates it from marasmus is the development of a generalized edema. The edema is a result of a very low level of intake of the essential amino acids, which causes the level of protein in the serum to fall to half or less than half of the normal values. The authors of this book studied marasmus and kwashiorkor among a sample of 32 Egyptian infants in 1966-1967 and concluded that no amount of nutritional health teaching could prevent kwashiorkor without an income level that would enable a family to afford an adequate diet.[23] It is possible that health teaching would have more effect in this country where kwashiorkor and marasmus are more sporadic events, but they still seem to be in part the result of poverty. Two brief case histories illustrate the problem:

> ... a one and one-half year old Navajo girl, brought to the hospital because of swelling, irritability, and loss of appetite of one week's duration. Parents considered her well until the onset of swelling. She had received "no milk for a long time" and had rarely been given meat. Diet consisted primarily of tea, soda water and beans.
> ... a two-year-old Navajo girl admitted because of sudden swelling. One month before a mild diarrhea began. [It] ceased two days prior to admission at which point the swelling occurred. Child had been increasingly listless. For the month during which there was diarrhea the child was fed nothing except soup and soda water and occasionally whole milk.[24]

If these case histories are typical examples it would seem that malnutrition in America is not only directly attributable to poverty but that it is also complicated by inadequate nutritional knowledge. Both of these children received soda pop. Many people fail to realize the low level of food value in such readily available and well-advertised foods such as soda pop, candy, potato chips, and sweetened breakfast cereals. And the persuasive powers of nutritionists are almost negligible compared to the influence exerted by advertising in the mass media.

It is, of course, very difficult to argue with hungry people if you are trying to dissuade them from eating. For generations hungry black children have eaten clay to fill their empty bellies and to stop the abdominal cramps which accompany hunger. A whole folk lore has grown up about clay eating until now there are people habituated to eating clay even when they are not hungry. Pregnant women with roots in the poor South often have strong desires for clay. They argue that it is particularly effective in combating the nausea of early pregnancy. Even today in some cities of the South, baked loaves of clay are hawked by street vendors. In the packed cities of the North where clay is usually not available many women have turned to laundry starch as a replacement—perhaps because it has a similar consistency. Clay has no food value, so unless it is comtaminated its ingestion causes no great harm. Laundry starch, on the other hand, is high in calories so that obesity can result, and since the clay and starch eaters are usually undernourished, obesity is coupled with an anemia as well as other signs of malnutrition. Because of the danger to mother and infant, public health nurses and nutritionists have for years argued against clay and starch eating. Recent research suggests, however, that the crucial factor in causing maternal and infant morbidity and mortality is the underlying malnutrition rather than the clay or starch themselves; the real problem then becomes one of supplying and teaching people to eat an adequate diet, and giving them the means to buy it.

As a result of the publicity given the first round of Senate hearings and the other hunger investigations, an official national nutritional survey was launched and preliminary findings were first issued in 1968. Arnold Schaefer, the director of the research, previously had done 34 nutrition studies in underdeveloped countries as a part of foreign aid and national defense efforts, and his finding of American malnutrition paralleled his other studies. He noted that malnutrition was a particularly serious problem in this country among young children. Poor children lagged behind their peers in physical development, in part because 34 percent were anemic, 33 percent suffered from a severe shortage of Vitamin A, and 16 percent had diets which lacked an adequate amount of Vitamin C.[25]

Hunger was also shown to be a serious problem among migrant workers, and hearings in 1969 by a new Senate committee under the chairmanship of George McGovern of South Dakota reported that most of the cattle and hogs in America were better fed and sheltered than the migrant families he visited in Florida. Migrant workers tend to be particularly disadvantaged because local officials seldom feel that they are a local responsibility.[26] But hunger seems to be everywhere. A California survey found that more than half of the 750,000 children in the state who were part of families receiving AFDC were required to live on incomes too low for their parents to purchase adequate diets.[27]

One of the most controversial yet serious consequences of malnutrition is the possible brain damage which it can cause. Although this sort of problem cannot be investigated in the political atmosphere of a Senate hearing, there is a substantial body of research knowledge related to this question. The negative consequences of inadequate nutrition start at least as early as the prenatal period, as undernutrition during pregnancy clearly effects reproductive outcomes. Recent research goes even further and suggests that nutritional status of the mother before pregnancy occurs is also important. The correlation of malnutrition and intellectual development is easiest to show by using prematurity as a factor linking the two. This is because prematurity is most likely to occur among groups whose socioeconomic status is low, and there is growing evidence that children who have birth weights below 2500 grams (5½ lb) tend to score lower on intelligence tests than those with higher birth weights.[28] A controlled study of 500 prematures born in Baltimore in 1952 matched with term infants on such factors as race, age, parity of mother, hospital, season of birth, and socioeconomic status showed that the premature infants were more intellectually retarded and more likely to have a physical or neurological problem when tested at ages three to five, six to seven, and eight to ten.[29]

Feeding the Hungry

In spite of the plethora of publicity and research on hunger which has been generated in the last few years, solutions to the problem have come slowly. At a White House conference on food and nutrition which was held in 1969 one of the participants summed up his feelings about the comparative volumes of talk and action's taking place by proposing a new slogan, "Let them eat rhetoric."

How to deal with hunger and malnutrition on a concrete level is a more serious problem. One of the more innovative solutions was adopted by H. Jack Geiger, a community health physician from Tufts Medical School, who established a clinic in Mound Bayou, Mississippi, in 1967 with funds from the Office of Economic Opportunity. Geiger realized that the most pressing medical problem faced by the poor people of the Mississippi delta was hunger. He felt that "pills without food were useless," so he stocked food in the pharmacy on the theory that "the specific treatment for malnutrition is food." Though health professionals have traditionally given dietary advice; dispensed protein, vitamin, and mineral supplements; and prescribed "formulas" for infants, they had considered bags of food as being more within the province of welfare workers. Geiger simply added food to the items that could be prescribed, and since the project was federally funded the hungry were given food as a part of their medical treatment. The results in increased health were impressive, although as a long-range solution to the problem the plan was not without problems, particularly those involving storage space in the pharmacy.[30]

When protests arose over this innovative interpretation of medication, the clinic workers, most of whom were local people, organized a cooperative farm with some 800 of the poorest families and then opened a cannery so that the summer's crops could be stored. The clinic workers went even further. While public health officials have traditionally emphasized the danger of contaminated wells and inadequate sanitary facilities, few turned to helping their constituency dig wells and build better privies as the Geiger group did. To enable physicians to make the best possible use of their talents, the Mound Bayou Clinic makes extensive use of public health nurses and indigenous aides who, in Geiger's words, compensate

> *for shortages of doctors, for helping interrupt the idiot revolving door game, the old business of diagnosing, treating, and sending a patient right back to the environment that produced his illness.*[31]

The experience of Geiger and the Mound Bayou workers suggests that to deal with poverty, health care might have to be interpreted more broadly. Since his experience, many others have begun to look upon hunger as a health problem.

Solution?

The agricultural act of 1949 stipulated that certain basic commodities bought under the price-support program could be distributed to the poor so that these materials would not be wasted. The program was extended in 1961 to allow more food items to be added to the list so that, presently, corn meal, corn grits, flour, nonfat dry milk, peanut butter, rice, rolled wheat, and 30 ounces of meat per person can be distributed each month. Although poultry, fruits, and vegetables are also purchased in quantity to support farm prices, in the past they have seldom been distributed to the poor.

Unfortunately also, counties have to decide whether they wish to participate in the commodity distribution programs, and the more impoverished county governments often decide they cannot afford the administrative costs involved in storing, transporting, and distributing the food. In 1967, for example, 331 of the 1,000 poorest counties had not yet applied for federal food assistance. To overcome this difficulty the Office of Economic Opportunity was authorized temporarily to distribute food on an emergency basis to "counteract conditions of starvation and malnutrition among the poor."[32] Unfortunately the emergency act was limited to temporary and small-scale efforts.

Even when a county does participate there are difficulties because eligibility is restricted to those receiving benefit from a federal- or state-aided public assistance program. States have differing standards and in some states a family of four with an annual income of $1800 is not eligible. Distribution points are often hard to reach, commodities are heavy (23 pounds per person), and distribution is usually on a monthly basis so that families without some means of private transportation are unable to get their food home. To correct some of the difficulties the food stamp program was also initiated so that low-income families could purchase food stamps at a discount instead of going to the food distribution center. The amount of stamps a family can buy and the purchase price they pay varies with the family income and the poor family has some choice in food selection. There are, however, difficulties in the program. It remains under the jurisdiction of the Department of Agriculture so that its goals are not clearly defined in terms of the needs of the hungry. This is because the Department of Agriculture is primarily concerned with the needs of farmers and the distribution of surplus farm commodities. Another problem is the fact that the program has failed to make provision for families with no income to buy stamps. Moreover, families with fixed expenses such as rent or pressing bills cannot afford to purchase the minimum they are required to buy if they are to use the stamps. Others are unable to get the specified amount of money together in one lump sum at a given date in the month. Most counties have been unwilling to allow for seasonal changes in income so that migrant farm workers cannot buy stamps in the summer because their income is too high and they cannot buy them in the winter because they lack money. The food stamp program is also administered through county governments and there are still counties which have refused the program because of administrative costs or other reasons.

Inevitably, because of the various problems involved in these programs, it is estimated that they reach only 18 percent of the poor or near poor.[33] The difficulties are exemplified by the school lunch program, which was conceived as a way to reach children with a good nutritional supplement as well as with nutritional education. Unfortunately, a 1967 survey found that approximately two-thirds of the six million children classed as living in poverty received no school lunch although somehow 20 million of the 50 million total population of school children were receiving lunches as part of the program. Investigation disclosed that the program actually served more children from the affluent suburbs than it did children from the rural or urban poverty areas. Again, the program is financed in a manner encouraging discrimination against the poor since the state was to put up three dollars for every dollar furnished by the federal government; this cut some states out, and in order to participate schools must have cafeterias, something which schools in poverty areas often lacked. Although federal guidelines were issued to broaden the school lunch program and to include more children in schools without kitchens and other poor children, the directive has not been effectively implemented because sufficient funds were never allocated to make this possible.[34]

Thus hunger remains a problem in our affluent society.[35] Although malnutrition is a serious problem for minority group members, it is found among all poverty populations whatever their ethnic identity. It remains somewhat more hidden but it is still an important factor linking poverty to less-than-optimum health.

Notes

1. Mollie Orshansky, "The Poverty Roster," in *Sources: A Blue Cross Report on the Health Problems of the Poor*, edited by Richard M. Ralston (Chicago, 1968), p. 10.
2. "The People Left Behind: The Rural Poor, A Report by the President's Commission on Rural Poverty," in *Poverty in America*, edited by Louis A. Ferman, Joyce L. Kornblugh, and Ann Haber (Ann Arbor: University of Michigan Press, revised edition, 1968), pp. 152-153.
3. *Ibid.*, p. 155.

4. United States Bureau of the Census, *Statistical Abstract of the United States,* 1970 (Washington, D.C.: U.S. Government Printing Office, 1970), p. 39; Table 47.
5. Rupert B. Vance, "The Region: A New Survey," in *The Southern Appalachian Region: A Survey*, edited by Thomas R. Ford (Lexington: University of Kentucky Press, 1962), pp. 4-5.
6. *Ibid.*, p. 7.
7. Jack E. Weller, *Yesterday's People: Life in Contemporary Appalachia* (Lexington: University of Kentucky Press, 1965); see also Harry M. Caudill, *Night Comes to the Cumberlands: A Biography of a Depressed Area* (Boston: Little, Brown and Co., 1963).
8. James S. Brown and George A. Hillery, Jr., "The Great Migration, 1940-60," in Ford, *op. cit.*, p. 54.
9. United States Bureau of the Census, *op. cit.*, p. 230; Tables 352 and 353.
10. United States Bureau of the Census, *Current Population Reports,* Series P-60, No. 76, "24 Million Americans — Poverty in the United States, 1969" (Washington, D.C.: U.S. Government Printing Office, 1970), p. 1.
11. California Legislative Assembly Committee on Health and Welfare, *Malnutrition: One Key to the Poverty Cycle* (January 1970), p. 13.
12. *Hunger, U.S.A.: A Report by the Citizens' Board of Inquiry into Hunger and Malnutrition in the United States* (Boston: Beacon Press, 1968), p. 11.
13. *Ibid.*, p. 3.
14. *Hearings Before the Subcommittee on Employment, Manpower and Poverty of the Committee on Labor and Public Welfare*, United States Senate, Ninetieth Congress, July 11 and 12, 1967 (Washington, D.C.: U.S. Government Printing Office), pp. 1-2.
15. *Ibid.*, pp. 4-62, *ad passim.*
16. *Ibid.*, pp. 63-106.
17. *Ibid.*, p. 188, and *Hunger, U.S.A.*, p. 194.
18. *Hunger, U.S.A.*, p. 19.
19. J. L. Filer, "The United States Today—Is It Free of Public Health Nutrition Problems Today—Anemia," presented to the American Public Health Association, Miami Beach, Fla., October 24, 1967, cited in *Hunger, U.S.A., op. cit.*
20. *Hunger, U.S.A., op. cit.*, p. 19.
21. C. B. Wolf, "Kwashiorkor on the Navaho Indian Reservation," U.S. Public Health Service, quoted in *Hunger, U.S.A.*, pp. 20-21.
22. Graciela Delgado, C. L. Brumback, and Mary Brice Deaver, "Eating Patterns Among Migrant Families," *Public Health Reports*, 76 (April 1961), pp. 349-355.
23. Bonnie Bullough, "Malnutrition among Egyptian Infants," *Nursing Research*, 18 (Spring 1969), p. 172.
24. Wolf, *op. cit.* Quoted in *Hunger, U.S.A.*, pp. 20-21.
25. Nick Kotz, *Let Them Eat Promises: The Politics of Hunger in America* (New York: Anchor Books, 1971), pp. 186-187.
26. *Hearings Before the Select Committee on Nutrition and Human Needs of the United States Senate*, Ninetieth Congress, Second Session, and Ninety-first Congress, Part 5B, Florida, Appendix (Washington, D.C.: U.S. Government Printing Office, 1969), p. 1835.
27. California Assembly Committee, *op. cit.*, pp. 1-26.

28. Herbert Birch and Joan Dye Gussow, *Disadvantaged Children: Health, Nutrition and School Failure* (New York: Harcourt, Brace, and World, 1970), pp. 123-153.
29. Hilda Knoch, R. Pasamanick, P. A. Harper, and R. Rider, "The Effect of Prematurity on Health and Growth," *American Journal of Public Health*, 49 (1959), pp. 1164-1173; Gerald Weiner, Rowland V. Rider, Wallace C. Oppel, Liselotte Fischer, and Paul A. Harper, "Correlates of Low Birth Weight: Psychological Status at Six to Seven Years of Age," *Pediatrics*, 35 (1965), pp. 434-444; G. Weiner, R. V. Rider, W. C. Oppel, and P. A. Harper, "Correlates of Low Birth Weight: Psychological Status at Eight to Ten Years of Age," *Pediatric Research*, 2 (March 1968), pp. 110-118.
30. Cynthia Kelly, "Health Care in the Mississippi Delta," *American Journal of Nursing*, 69 (April 1969), pp. 759-763.
31. *Ibid.*
32. *Hunger, U.S.A., op. cit.*, pp. 55-56.
33. *Ibid.*, p. 50.
34. Nick Kotz, *op. cit.*, pp. 55, 227.
35. *White House Conference on Food, Nutrition and Health*, Final Report, Chairman: Jean Mayer (Washington, D.C.: U.S. Government Printing Office, 1970).

7

Mental Health and Mental Illness

A dominant theme of this book has been that both poverty and ethnic identity need to be considered in any explanation of minority health problems. This is as true of mental health as it is of physical health. Nevertheless, some words of caution have to be given. This is true because there has always been a tendency to blame the ills of society on the poor—to indicate that the poor are poor because they are feeble, less able, or mentally ill. This is the implication of an 1856 report which stated that the "pauper class" in Massachusetts "furnished proportionately sixty four times as many cases of insanity as the independent class."[1] While there is a correlation between mental illness and socioeconomic status, the relationship is a complex one which has only begun to become evident through the research of the last 30 or 40 years.

A pioneering study in the field, done in Chicago by Robert E. L. Faris and H. Warren Dunham, was published in 1939. The two investigators found that patients who were diagnosed as schizophrenic were most likely to have home addresses near the central part of the city—in the slum and rooming house neighborhoods—while patients who were diagnosed as manic depressive were scattered throughout the whole city. Since schizophrenia was the most common type of functional psychosis, the high rate of this disease found in poverty neighborhoods helped account for the correlation between hospitalization and low socioeconomic status. In trying to explain their findings, Faris and Dunham hypothesized that schizophrenia might be more common in poverty neighborhoods because people in such areas felt a greater sense of isolation owing to the social disorganization of their neighborhood.[2] This interpretation touched off a lively debate that is still going on. On the one hand, researchers have found that slums are not particularly disorganized, only that their social structure is different from that of the more affluent neighborhoods.[3] On the other hand, and much more basically, the interpretation has been challenged because it implies a causal chain between poverty and schizophrenia. Later researchers, including Dunham himself, have argued that poverty might be a consequence of schizophrenia rather than its cause. The schizophrenic individual may drift down to live in a poor neighborhood because of the socially debilitating symptoms of his illness.[4]

Since the possible explanations have such great social consequences, the research has become voluminous. In a review of 44 major empirical studies investigating the relationship of socioeconomic status and psychological disorders, Bruce and Barbara Dohrenwend found that in spite of differences in design, the vast majority of studies reported that psychological disorders were more common among poor people than among middle- or upper-class individuals. Usually it was the lowest class or stratum, no matter how defined, which had the largest population of the mentally ill. They concluded that although the interpretations of the data might be subject to debate there could be little quarrel with the basic correlation between poverty and psychological disorders.[5]

The Complexity of the Problem

The causes of this correlation is still being investigated. A methodological problem inherent in the research is how to define mental illness. A New Haven study, started in 1950 by a team of sociologists and psychiatrists headed by August Hollingshead and

Fredrick Redlich, used diagnosed illness to define operationally what they meant by a psychiatric disorder. To find their sample they contacted all of the mental hospitals, private psychiatrists, and clinics in the area for patients diagnosed as having mental illness. They then classified the residents of New Haven into five social classes, a not particularly difficult thing to do since New Haven, the home of Yale University, had already been the subject of several studies of class structure. They again found that the poor people were more likely to be diagnosed as having some type of psychiatric disorder than those who were richer—due, they believed, to the stress of living in a lower-class environment. They found that there were significant differences, depending upon a person's social class, in the type of diagnosis given. Psychoses, for example, were more commonly diagnosed among the two lowest of the five classes while neuroses were more often found among the top three classes. The finding is not so clear-cut as it might seem since it could mean either that the stress of poverty produced more serious types of mental illness, or it could also suggest that psychotherapists are more likely to diagnose an illness as a neurosis if the patient is from the middle or upper class, but will call it a psychosis if the patient comes from a lower social class.[6]

The New Haven study was also criticized because it included only diagnosed illness. A midtown Manhattan study under the direction of Leo Srole and another team of psychiatrists and sociologists attempted to broaden the definition of mental illness to include persons not under treatment. They gathered data by means of a lengthy interview in which a random sample of people in different strata of society indicated their own feelings and problems. Their mental health status was determined by their answers to the questions. This procedure made the incidence of mental illness seem much higher because it included all of the untreated cases, but the proportion of disorders was still highest among the lowest social stratum. In an attempt to determine whether poverty was the cause or consequence of these symptoms, the investigators looked also at the social class of the parents of the people they interviewed. Although they did find that those persons whose parents were of low social class were more likely to report symptoms or be diagnosed as ill, the individual's own social class was more strongly related to the probability of his having a mental disorder than that of his parents. Mental illness, in fact, occurred more often among the people who were downwardly mobile than those who moved up the social scale during their lifetime.[7]

In a sense we are back to the original findings of Faris and Dunham, but still without any degree of certainty. The main reason for replication of studies and cautious concern about the link between socioeconomic status and psychiatric disorders is that researchers are still unsure about the cause of many mental illnesses. The studies linking poverty and mental illness suggest there is a sociogenic relationship. Psychiatrists, following the lead of Sigmund Freud, have customarily attributed most symptoms of mental illness to stress of early childhood experiences and problems in family interactions. In turn they have tended to discount most of the later stresses which sociologists feel are so important. A more recent trend, particularly in the research about schizophrenia, has been to reemphasize the role of biological determinants, particularly possible genetic causes. Several studies in which twins were utilized as research subjects have raised questions about the nature of schizophrenia. It has been found that a schizophrenic monozygotic twin is more likely to have a twin who is afflicted than a schizophrenic whose twin is not identical. These findings are also supported by other family surveys which reinforce the concept that there is a hereditary tendency to develop the disease.[8] Nevertheless, most authorities still believe that there are also environmental influences in the development of schizophrenia. A comparison with tuberculosis is often made because tuberculosis is both an organic disease and an environmental disease. Similarly, schizophrenia now seems to be caused by a combination of biological, social, and psychological elements, with poverty implicated as one of the crucial social elements in this causal chain.[9]

The unwillingness to discard the factor of environment is in part due to the fact that it enters into the mental health picture in so many other ways. The New Haven survey mentioned above had a 10-year follow-up study of the patients identified as mentally ill in the initial study. In this research it was found that people received a different type of treatment depending upon their social-class position. Middle- and upper-class patients were more likely to have received psychotherapy or somatotherapy and were able to be cared for on an out-patient basis or in a doctor's office. Their families were not only better able to pay for the therapy but they were also more willing to tolerate the ill person at home—either because they had more ample housing or could hire outside help if needed. Lower-class patients, on the other hand, had seldom received any effective therapy. They were more likely to have been committed to a long-term public facility where they received little more than custodial care mingled with some drug therapy. They drifted into chronic mental illness, disappearing into the back wards of the state mental hospitals.[10] These differences in treatment patterns are important in explaining the higher overall percentage of mental illness among people with low incomes, regardless of the position one takes on the causality of mental illness. Most experts agree that the present state of psychotherapy leaves much to be desired but that it is still the most effective treatment modality developed to date. At the crowded mental hospitals, where most of the poor end up, there are so few psychotherapists that the care offered must be classed as primarily custodial.

Tied in with this finding is the nature of long-term hospitalization itself. Erving Goffman believes that long-term hospitalization in a total institution such as a mental hospital actually causes people to behave in peculiar ways. The stress begins with the admission procedures themselves, which strip the patient of his individual identity. In order to cope with his inmate status the patient then develops either an apathetic posture or takes on some special, peculiar coping mechanism which makes him seem not quite sane. What is diagnosed as psychopathology can well be a realistic response to the hospitalization experience. This means that the individual who is admitted to a mental hospital, particularly one of the larger public institutions, is at a marked disadvantage in comparison to the person who can be treated in his accustomed surroundings.[11]

Finances are not the only barrier between lower-class patients and psychotherapists. Psychiatrists, clinical psychologists, and psychiatric social workers tend to be recruited almost exclusively from middle- and upper-class backgrounds, and until recently the only ethnic minority well represented in the group were Jews. Since this is the case it is possible that therapists are afflicted with a certain amount of class and racial ethnocentrism.

This prejudice is clearly evident in the types of patients whom the psychotherapists chose for therapy. It has been shown, for example, that they tend to avoid patients whose education has been meager or whose occupations are unskilled. Such exclusion is justified on the grounds that the lower-class patient cannot verbalize adequately or that he does not have the necessary cognitive skills to participate in the therapeutic process. This is undoubtedly true but the same type of statement can be made about children and psychotherapists have found ways to deal with youngsters. It seems rather that the psychotherapists do not feel the same empathy for the problems of the lower-class patients that they do for those patients whose problems are similar to their own. Unfortunately, this generalization tends to be true even for those few therapists whose origins were lower-middle class or lower-class. This means that psychotherapy, in or out of the hospital, is simply not available to most poor or minority patients.[1][2]

Ethnic Identity and Mental Illness

It is not only the relationship of poverty and mental illness which is a matter of debate, but even more controversial is the relationship of ethnic identity to the incidence of psychoses and neuroses. Much of the difficulty comes from the fact that there is considerably more polemics than hard research in the field. Writers from the "right" try to prove that one group is inferior to another while writers from the "left" argue that the present social structure needs reform. Although we would fall into the second category, it seems obvious that the most effective reforms should be based upon objective findings. Unfortunately the evidence is not at all clear since, as Benjamin Pasamanick pointed out, most of the investigators in the past have demonstrated bias either in the collection of the data or in its interpretation. The controversy in the United States goes back at least to the census of 1840, which found that the rates of institutionalization for Negroes was higher in the North than in the South. Advocates of slavery immediately interpreted this as meaning that the innately inferior Negroes fared better under slavery than they did living as free men in the North. Ignored in the polemics was the fact that the South had fewer institutions than the North and that the institution of slavery itself could afford to be somewhat tolerant of certain kinds of mental disorder that induce greater submission. Moreover, the South was much more rural than the North and it is in the urban centers where the mentally ill were most likely to be institutionalized. However, the same kind of conclusion appeared in some of the studies in 1880 when there was growing hostility toward immigrants, particularly the Irish Catholics. The official census report of that year stated that there was an "extraordinary ratio of insanity among the foreign born."[13]

As we try to escape the biases of the past, however, we still must report that Negro admission rates are higher in the mental hospitals in proportion to population,[14] and Negroes stay longer in the hospital than do white patients. How much is this an indication of racial predisposition and how much is due to poverty? When socioeconomic status is carefully controlled, psychosis rates among Negroes and whites appear to be similar. This implies that the higher rates of hospitalization are due more to poverty than to any ethnic identity.[15] Of some eight studies collected by the Dohrenwends to compare the rates of psychological disorders among Negro and white populations, four report higher rates for Negroes and four report higher rates for whites. The evidence is even more contradictory than this brief summary would indicate. The Dohrenwends, themselves, for example, found a high incidence of self-reported psychiatric symptoms among Puerto Ricans in New York City and a low incidence for Negroes.[16] In Texas, E. Gartly Jace found a lower incidence of diagnosed psychoses among the Spanish-surname population than among either Anglos or nonwhites.[17] The only thing one can conclude from the available evidence is that there is at present no proven correlation between ethnic identity and the type of psychoses such as schizophrenia in which an individual loses contact with reality.

Personality Damage

These findings do not mean, however, that there are not much more subtle correlations between race and poverty and mental illness. In fact the most serious mental health consequence of minority status might well be the damage which poverty and discrimination inflict on the attitudes and intellectual development of the growing child. Generations of researchers have found that both race and socioeconomic status correlate significantly with all of the common measurements of intelligence.[18] Moreover, the effects of both race and socioeconomic status tend, at least at times, to be additive. This is evidenced by the fact that in many studies of intelligence poor white children score higher than poor black children but neither group scores as well as families with adequate incomes.

Complicating the nature of the findings is another argument between nature versus nurture. Arthur Jensen was able to shake the scholarly world of educational psychology a few years ago when he made a strong case for the genetic determinants of I.Q. Jensen believed that compensatory education was a failure and the reason it had failed was because educators had neglected to take account of the importance of the genetic factor in predicting intelligence levels. He suggested that there might well be inherited racial and social-class differences in ability that doomed all such educational efforts to failure.[19] Jensen became the focus of a sharp controversy because many people felt that he was trying to revive racist ideologies about superior and inferior races. Certainly Jensen tended to lend support to some of the racist arguments, but what is needed either to prove or disprove his assertions is more serious biological research.[20] Until such evidence is forthcoming the debate is more or less meaningless. Most authorities agree that regardless of biological potential, environmental factors still play a crucial role in fostering or hindering intellectual achievement. It is also important to realize that environmental stresses can have biological consequences. As has been reported in earlier chapters, such factors as severe malnutrition, prematurity, and accidents at delivery—all of which are most associated with low socioeconomic status—can have lasting negative consequences for mental development.

Unfortunately, as the child grows, disadvantages associated with poverty and ethnicity tend to be cumulative so that he falls farther and farther behind in relationship to his peer group. This process can be observed in almost any school where there are children from poverty backgrounds. The child from such a background tends to come to school with cognitive deficits because of his less-favorable preschool experiences; he has probably seen fewer books, traveled less, had fewer verbal interchanges, and so on. The Head Start program was aimed at trying to supply some of these experiences by broadening the child's horizons, but it is doubtful whether two years of Head Start can make up for neglect and lack of opportunity before and after nursery school. In school itself the comparative lack of experience and supportive action at home helps cause the child to fail in the early grades. This is most likely to happen if the child also has intestinal parasites or is malnourished. With these early failures his self-confidence is impaired. School becomes an unpleasant experience so that there is little motivation for achievement. These factors reinforce each other as low achievement leads to low grades and lack of positive reinforcement from the teacher leads to a further loss of self-esteem.[21]

Teacher expectations also enter into this picture, furthering the process since it is a truism that people tend to act as they are expected to act. A teacher, often on what seems to him to be quite reasonable grounds, may be convinced that children from minority and poverty backgrounds do not learn as fast or behave as well as children from more advantaged backgrounds. The results of such attitudes were demonstrated effectively in an elementary school in northern California where both teachers and pupils were unknowing guinea pigs. Students in all eighteen classes of the school were given a standard battery of intelligence tests which the teachers were led to believe had predictive value for identifying future "academic blooming." Unknown to the teachers, the researchers then chose a random sample of about 20 percent of the children from each classroom and told the teachers that these children could be expected to show a burst of achievement. The teachers were also told to keep this information to themselves and not tell the students. All the children were tested again at four- and eight-month intervals, and a teacher rating was done on each of the students at the end of the year. The results were just as the teachers thought the tests had predicted. The randomly selected academic bloomers bloomed. They were rated by their teachers as more interesting, curious, happy, and more likely to become successful in the future. These students also showed a more rapid gain on intelligence-test scores, particularly in their ability to reason, than did their classmates.[22] The experiment demonstrated how crucial the attitudes of teachers were in determining success.

In addition to the cognitive and verbal deficits which accompany low socioeconomic status, the child with a minority identity also starts school with other disadvantages. By the age of five or six he often has developed feelings of racial prejudice against himself. The present black power movement has proclaimed in a strident voice that "black is beautiful." This is an essential first step in developing a confident self-identity, but it will only be effective when it becomes an accepted statement rather than a battle cry. It will be even better when it does not have to be said at all because black children will know that they are beautiful just as white children know, for the most part, that they are beautiful. That day has not yet come. In spite of widespread popular beliefs that children do not know prejudice, a series of studies done by Kenneth and Mamie Clark found that preschool children were not only aware of their own racial identity but that they had already acquired positive and negative feelings about that identity. The Clarks tested these feelings by presenting children with dolls of differing skin shades or having them color pictures with crayons. Quite consistently Negro children chose light skins as more desirable and attractive. Their comments indicated that they had not only learned that they were Negroes but they were well aware of and believed in the negative stereotypes that accompanied such an identity.[23] The findings of other researchers have supported those of the Clarks. In sociometric tests in which children were asked to select the child in their class they would most like to play with or sit next to, both white and Negro children tend to select white children.[24] The denial of self as psychologically or physically beautiful was dramatically demonstrated one year in the early 1950s when the Negro newspaper, *The Chicago Defender*, unwittingly selected a white girl who was passing as a Negro as their beauty queen. The reasons for the choice were obvious: she had the fewest Negroid features of any of the candidates. Fortunately, the "black is beautiful" movement is working to change these stereotypes among young women, and in fact, some Negro girls whose hair is not particularly curly are now putting it up into tight pin curls each night in order to achieve the proper Afro look.

The custom of human beings to search for their self-identity in the reflected image of others[25] places any despised minority group at a disadvantage when it comes to raising mentally healthy children. This is why racial prejudice has such serious consequences for mental health. Though there is little research about the evaluation of self that is made by Puerto Rican or Mexican-American children, it would seem that there would be similar forces at work as among Negroes, although perhaps not so severe. It is possible for the Puerto Rican to return to Puerto Rico and the Mexican-American to visit Mexico to find a conscious self-identity, a feeling which in the past has been denied to the Negro.

Segregated schools also reinforce feelings of inferiority. In his comprehensive study of educational opportunities undertaken for the United States Office of Education, James Coleman concluded that segregated schools were very damaging to minority children. His team measured three types of attitudes related to academic motivation: (1) an interest in school work, (2) self-concept regarding ability, and (3) a sense of control over one's own rewards. He found all three factors were related to academic achievement, but the most crucial was the third factor, control over one's own fate. Negro children who felt the most powerless were the least likely to do well in school. As the proportion of white students in the school enrollment increased, the Negro student felt better able to cope with the dominant white world and both his feelings of control and his educational achievement increased.[26] Unfortunately, the feelings of powerlessness which develop out of segregated experiences have long-range consequences. In the Los Angeles study of housing segregation carried out by one of the authors of this book it was found that the feelings of alienation, including powerlessness and anomie, kept even successful middle-class Negroes from making the effort to move to an integrated neighborhood although they placed value on this kind of residence. The ghetto in effect builds its own walls because the feelings of alienation of the adults were more strongly related to childhood experiences with segregated schools and neighborhoods than to childhood economic deprivation.[27]

The apathy, the alienation, and the negative self-image created by poverty, prejudice, and discrimination carry over to health in both direct and indirect ways. If mental health is defined positively as a sense of psychic well-being rather than just the absence of certain debilitating behavioral symptoms, the person who has low self-esteem or who feels that he has no power over his own fate rates low on a continuum of mental health. More importantly, feelings of hopelessness and powerlessness act as barriers to people seeking preventive health care because planning seems useless. Thus they are more likely to develop preventable physical illness and to wait until their illness has progressed so far that they require long-term hospitalization. These negative feelings also fit into other causal sequences which have consequences for health. The child whose achievement in school is blocked by his social-class background or his minority status is likely to drop out of school before he is able to gain a useful occupational skill; this means that his later employment is marginal. The cycle then continues as he is unable to furnish a good environment for his children or to buy good health care in a society in which health care is a commodity to be bought, and the complex Gordian knot becomes even more impossible to unravel.

Anger

Apathy and withdrawal are the consequences of economic and racial discrimination; anger is still another. The psychiatrists, William Grier and Price Cobbs, have described an ever-present, gut-level rage as the outstanding race-related phenomenon they see in their black patients.[28] In the past, fear of violent reprisals and the conditioning for apathy and powerlessness had forced most Negroes to suppress overt expression of rage. However, as these barriers have begun to be dismantled, open violence has erupted. The race riots of the 19th and early 20th centuries differed significantly from the current ones in that the earlier ones were instigated by white gangs who invaded black neighborhoods and attacked the residents while the current ones are often instigated by blacks.[29] The 1935 Harlem and the 1943 Detroit riots originated in the Negro ghettoes and were aimed at white-owned property. It was not until the decade of the 1960s, however, that Negro rioting reached almost epidemic proportion and focused public attention on the problem of ghetto living.

To study the riots, President Lyndon B. Johnson appointed the National Advisory Commission on Civil Disorders. The commission, somewhat to the surprise of most of its liberal critics, reported that the basic cause of the riots was white racism. This racism, translated into discrimination, caused large numbers of Negroes to feel angry, frustrated, and cut-off from any legitimate outlet. To solve the problems the commission advised basic reforms in the administration of justice, the opening-up of employment, housing, and educational opportunities, and a full-scale effort to lessen the level of frustration in the ghetto.[30] In 1970 and 1971 there were similar outbreaks of violence in the Mexican-American barrios of Los Angeles, with similar root causes.

From a mental health standpoint it could be argued that the open expression of this rage is a healthier response than the continued forced repression, although from the standpoint of public policy the riots are no solution. It is interesting to note that while most ghetto residents understood and sympathized with the riots usually only from 10 to 20 percent actively participated in them.[31] In effect most people continued to control or repress their anger with the system. Repression of anger, however, shows up in other ways. It has been argued that one of the consequences of this type of control of pent-up anger is high blood pressure. Though few large-scale studies on the subject have been carried out, the fact that the rate of essential hypertension is much higher among the Negro population than among the white is suggestive of such a possibility.[32]

Suicide, Alcoholism, and Drug Addiction

Also unclear is the correlation of race and suicide. Even the statistics which relate socioeconomic status to suicide are not always consistent. Using data from England, Louis Dublin found more suicides among the highest and the lowest social classes.[33] In most American studies a more simple correlation between low socioeconomic status and suicide has been found.[34] Nevertheless, most authorities hold that sex and race are more significant than income when it comes to predicting suicide, although the psychodynamics and the precipitating cause of suicide tend to vary from one group to another. For example, more men than women kill themselves and the stress which triggers their suicide tends to be work-related while those women who destroy themselves are more often disturbed by marital or family problems.[35]

The epidemic proportion of suicide and suicide-related behavior among Indians was pointed out in an earlier chapter. In order to explain this high rate, researchers turned to the concept of anomie originated by Durkheim.[36] In effect, rapid social and cultural change have left the Indians without the societal underpinnings which usually constrain people from committing suicide. The same explanation seems to account for the high rates among the foreign-born Americans since immigrants are similarly cut-off from the environment in which social norms were more stable and family relationships more available. Foreign-born males have a suicide rate that is almost double that of the population as a whole, while foreign-born females have a rate that is 74 percent higher than the female average.[37]

Contrary to expectations, however, suicide rates are not high among the major American ethnic minority populations. Negroes and Mexican-Americans have low suicide rates. Residents of the United States born in Mexico, for example, have the lowest rate of any group of immigrants: 7.9 per hundred thousand in 1960 compared to the national average of 10.6 for that year. Even lower is the general nonwhite ratio (including Negroes) of 4.5 per hundred thousand. Since most of the groups classed as nonwhite, including Orientals and Indians, have higher-than-average suicide rates, the Negro rate must be judged as very low.[38]

Suicide statistics, however, are misleading because what constitutes suicide is dependent upon what various officials define as suicide. In general, suicide is more likely to be reported in the North than in the South and in urban areas than in rural areas. What constitutes suicide can also be debated; this causes difficulty not only for theorists but also for individuals who must decide as a part of their official duties whether an individual did or did not kill himself. To many people suicide represents an escape from intolerable loneliness or the overwhelming problems of life.[39] Escape is also possible through drugs or alcohol, so that it has been argued that alcoholism and drug addiction can also be forms of suicidal behavior.[40] Obviously such a conceptualization of suicide would change the statistical picture for minority group members.

There is, for example, a fairly high rate of problem drinking among Negroes,[41] and such drinking patterns can be a factor in accidental deaths and cirrhosis of the liver or they can complicate other types of illnesses. The narcotizing effect of alcoholism is one way of dealing with frustration and helping one to escape from painful realities. Drinking is not confined to lower socioeconomic groups and it seems also to be common among middle-status Negroes.[42]

Most studies of drug addiction report that chronic users are likely to originate in the poorest neighborhoods and be members of minority groups. Addiction is rare in rural areas; it tends to be concentrated in the urban slums and within these areas the users tend to come from the most miserable circumstances. Addiction, in fact, correlates highly with almost any form of human misery including poverty, unemployment, broken homes, low education levels, and substandard housing. Even with these common background factors, researchers are finding that no single explanatory principle can completely account for the high incidence of narcotic use in the urban slums. People start using drugs for a variety of reasons, including feelings of failure, alienation, or emptiness.[43] Then they continue with drug use to avoid withdrawal symptoms[44] or because the drug subculture gives them a way of life. Narcotics, which are readily available in the poverty neighborhoods, become an answer to feelings of hopelessness and frustration that otherwise seem to have no answer.

There are, however, changes in the patterns of drug usage, particularly when it comes to the hallucinogenic drugs, the barbiturates, and marijuana, which have been adopted by a broader youth culture. At the present time, marijuana smokers are likely to come from higher-income families with better educated parents. Probably in the period before 1960 the average marijuana user would have been black, lived in an urban slum, and suffered socioeconomic discrimination.[45] The hallucinogenic drugs and barbiturates, on the other hand, had their beginnings with the youth culture rather than with the poverty population. Although deaths are common among barbiturate users, the opiates are more debilitating, and they remain the most common drug problem among minority group members.

From this brief survey, it seems evident that the association of poverty and ethnic identity to mental illness is a complex one. The relationship between low socioeconomic status and the psychoses is clear, but diagnostic and treatment differences may be the reason for this correlation. Poverty and discrimination are obviously implicated as causal factors in school failures and in the creation of a ghetto attitude which is marked on one hand by an apathetic withdrawal and on the other hand by a bubbling anger which can break through in a violent revolt. The Indian minority has a high suicide rate, but Negroes, Puerto Ricans, and Mexican-Americans are less likely to be victims of suicide, unless the anesthetizing destruction of alcoholism and drug addiction are defined as suicide.

Notes

1. Myron G. Sandifer, Jr. "Social Psychiatry A Hundred Years Ago," *American Journal of Psychiatry*, 118 (February 1962), pp. 749-750.
2. Robert E. L. Faris and H. Warren Dunham, *Mental Disorders in Urban Areas: An Ecological Study of Schizophrenia and Other Psychoses* (Chicago: University of Chicago Press, 1939).
3. Gerald D. Suttles, *The Social Order of the Slum: Ethnicity and Territory in the Inner City* (Chicago: University of Chicago Press, 1968).
4. H. Warren Dunham, *Community and Schizophrenia: An Epidemiological Analysis* (Detroit: Wayne State University Press, 1965).
5. Bruce P. Dohrenwend and Barbara Snell Dohrenwend, *Social Status and Psychological Disorder: A Causal Inquiry* (New York: Wiley-Interscience, 1969), pp. 10-19.
6. August B. Hollingshead and Fredrick C. Redlich, "Social Stratification and Psychiatric Disorders," *American Sociological Review*, 18 (April 1953), pp. 163-169; August B. Hollingshead and Fredrick C. Redlich, *Social Class and Mental Illness* (New York: John Wiley and Sons, 1958).
7. Leo Srole, Thomas S. Langner, Stanley T. Michael, Marvin K. Opler, and Thomas C. Rennie, *Mental Health in the Metropolis: The Midtown Manhattan Study*, vol. 1 (New York: McGraw-Hill), 1962.
8. Leonard L. Heston, "The Genetics of Schizophrenia and Schizoid Disease," *Science*, 167 (January 1970), pp. 249-256; Dohrenwend and Dohrenwend, *op. cit.*, pp. 32-38.
9. Rema LaPouse, Mary A. Monk, and Milton Terris, "The Drift Hypothesis and Socio-Economic Differentials in Schizophrenia," *American Journal of Public Health*, 46 (August 1956), pp. 978-986.
10. Jerome K. Myers and Lee L. Bean in collaboration with Max P. Pepper, *A Decade Later: A Follow-Up of Social Class and Mental Illness* (New York: John Wiley), 1968.
11. Erving Goffman, *Asylums: Essays on the Social Situation of Mental Patients and Other Inmates* (New York: Anchor Books, 1961).

12. David W. Rowden, Jerry B. Michel, Ronald C. Dillehay, and Harry W. Martin, "Judgments About Candidates for Psychotherapy: The Influence of Social Class and Insight-Verbal Ability," *Journal of Health and Social Behavior*, 11 (March 1970), pp. 51-58.
13. Benjamin Pasamanick, "A Survey of Mental Disease in an Urban Population," in *Mental Health and Segregation*, edited by Martin M. Grossack (New York: Springer, 1963), pp. 150-157.
14. David C. Wilson and Edna M. Lantz, "Cultural Change and Negro State Hospital Admission," in Grossack, *op. cit.*, pp. 139-149.
15. Pasamanick, *op. cit.*
16. Dohrenwend and Dohrenwend, *op. cit.*, pp. 13-16.
17. E. Gartly Jaco, "Mental Health of the Spanish-American in Texas," in *Culture and Mental Health: Cross Cultural Studies*, edited by Marvin Opler (New York: The Macmillan Company, 1959), pp. 467-485.
18. Thomas F. Pettigrew, *A Profile of the Negro American* (Princeton, N.J.: D. Van Nostrand, 1964), pp. 100-135; Martin Whiteman and Martin Deutsch, "Social Disadvantage as Related to Intellective and Language Development," in *Social Class, Race and Psychological Development*, edited by Martin Deutsch, Irwin Katz, and Arthur R. Jensen (New York: Holt, Rinehart & Winston, 1968), pp. 86-114.
19. Arthur R. Jensen, "How Much Can We Boost I.Q. and Scholastic Achievement?" *Harvard Educational Review*, 39 (Winter 1969), pp. 1-123. The controversy between Jensen and other scholars is well presented in the issues of the *Harvard Educational Review* which followed this presentation.
20. I. I. Gottesman, "Biogenetics of Race and Class," in *Social Class, Race and Psychological Development, op. cit.*, pp. 11-51.
21. Martin Whiteman and Martin Deutsch, *op. cit.*
22. Robert Rosenthal and Lenore Jacobson, "Self Fulfilling Prophesies in the Classroom: Teacher's Expectations as Unintended Determinants of Pupils' Intellectual Competence," in *Social Class, Race and Psychological Development, op. cit.*, pp. 219-253; Robert Rosenthal and Lenore Jacobson, *Pygmalion in the Classroom: Teacher Expectation and Pupils' Intellectual Development* (New York: Holt, Rinehart & Winston, 1969).
23. Kenneth B. Clark, *Prejudice and Your Child* (Boston: The Beacon Press, 1955) and Kenneth and Mamie Clark, "Emotional Factors in Racial Identification and Preference in Negro Children," in *Mental Health and Segregation, op. cit.*, pp. 53-63.
24. Harold Proshansky and Peggy Newton, "The Nature and Meaning of Negro Self-Identity," in *Social Class, Race and Psychological Development, op. cit.*, pp. 178-218. This article includes a comprehensive review of such studies.
25. *The Social Psychology of George Herbert Mead*, edited by Anselm Strauss (Chicago: University of Chicago Press, 1956).
26. James S. Coleman, Ernest Q. Campbell, Carol Hobson, James McPartland, Alexander Mood, Frederic Weinfield, and Robert Jork, *Equality of Educational Opportunity* (Washington, D.C.: U.S. Office of Education, 1966).
27. Bonnie Bullough, *Social Psychological Barriers to Housing Desegregation* (Los Angeles: University of California, Housing, Real Estate and Urban Land Studies Program, 1969) and Bonnie Bullough, "Alienation and

School Segregation, *Integrated Education*, in press, 1972.

28. William H. Grier and Price M. Cobbs, *Black Rage* (New York: Basic Books, 1968).
29. William M. Tuttle, Jr., *Race Riot* (New York: Atheneum, 1970).
30. Otto Kerner, Chairman, *Report of the National Advisory Commission on Civil Disorders* (Washington, D.C.: U.S. Government Printing Office, 1968).
31. Kerner, *op. cit.*, pp. 73-77; Robert M. Fogelson and Robert B. Hill, "Who Riots? A Study of Participation in the 1967 Riots," in *Supplemental Studies for the National Advisory Commission on Civil Disorders*, Chairman, Otto Kerner (Washington, D.C.: U.S. Government Printing Office, 1968), p. 223.
32. V. E. Schulz and E. H. Schwab, "Arteriolar Hypertension in the American Negro," *American Heart Journal*, 11 (January 1963), pp. 66-74; George Getz, "High Blood Pressure - The Unknown Killer," *The Los Angeles Times* (Report of Papers Read at the American Heart Association Convention, 1971), Los Angeles, November 12, 1971.
33. Louis I. Dublin, *Suicide: A Sociological and Statistical Study* (New York: Ronald Press, 1963), pp. 61-65.
34. Ronald W. Maris, *Social Forces in Urban Suicide* (Homewood, Ill., The Dorsey Press, 1969), p. 160.
35. Warren Breed, "Suicide, Migration and Race: A Study of Cases in New Orleans," *The Journal of Social Issues*, 22 (January 1966), pp. 30-43.
36. Emile Durkheim, *Suicide: A Study in Sociology*, translated by John A. Spaulding and George Simpson (Glencoe, Ill.: The Free Press, 1957), pp. 241-276.
37. Dublin, *op. cit.*, p. 31.
38. *Ibid.*, Tables II, X, XI, pp. 211, 216, 21-19; Breed, *op. cit.;* Sanford Labovits, "Variation in Suicide Rates," in *Suicide*, edited by Jack P. Gibbs (New York: Harper & Row, 1968), pp. 57-73.
39. For a discussion of the various meanings of suicide see Jack Douglas, *The Social Meaning of Suicide* (Princeton: Princeton University Press, 1967).
40. Karl A. Menninger, *Man Against Himself* (New York: Harcourt, Brace & Company, 1938).
41. George L. Maddox, "Drinking Among Negroes: Inferences from the Drinking Patterns of Selected Negro Male Collegians," *Journal of Health and Social Behavior*, 8 (June 1967), pp. 114-120.
42. E. Franklin Frazier, *Black Bourgeoisie* (New York: Collier Books, 1962), p. 190.
43. Isadore Chein, "Psychological, Social and Epidemiological Factors in Drug Addiction," in *Rehabilitating the Narcotic Addict*, a Report of the Institute on New Developments in the Rehabilitation of the Narcotic Addict (Washington, D.C.: U.S. Government Printing Office, 1966), pp. 53-66.
44. Alfred R. Lindesmith, "Basic Problems in the Social Psychology of Addiction and a Theory," in *Narcotic Addiction*, edited by John A. O'Donnell and John C. Ball (New York: Harper & Row, 1966), pp. 91-109.
45. Erich Goode, *The Marijuana Smokers* (New York: Basic Books, 1970), pp. 35-39.

8

Discrimination and Segregation

In the 20th century, American medicine has been regarded as an occupation for the upper-middle classes. Costly and time-consuming education has made it difficult if not impossible for a poor person to become a high-status health professional. In fact, with only slight exaggeration, it can be argued that until the advent of the GI Bill in the aftermath of World War II, college education itself was primarily a middle-class phenomenon. Since those students who continued their studies beyond the bachelor's degree had to have even greater economic resources, the fact that physicians came from the more affluent sections of society seems self-explanatory. As late as 1961 some 40 percent of all medical students came from families whose income was in the top 8 percent of the population.[1]

In a sense medicine was not particularly different from other professional occupations in its educational demands, but in another sense it was much more elitist in orientation because, unlike law or college teaching, medicine demanded that the training be taken in a concentrated dose, and the long hours of duty and study made it difficult for the would-be physician to have a part-time job on the side. It is true that there were occasional scholarships, and that in spite of all obstacles some students from a poverty background made it through medical school. However, to do so required greater intelligence and dedication than that demonstrated by the average medical student; the less affluent student also needed better luck and a devoted family since not only he had to sacrifice but his whole family as well. The very structure of medical training was designed to exclude almost all but the more well-to-do.

Medical schools were also geographically concentrated, and in fact until after World War II many states and regions were without medical schools. This meant that it was necessary for the would-be student to relocate in an area far from home and to maintain a second household, a task which added to his economic burdens. Dentistry, if only because the course of studies was shorter and the entrance requirements less rigorous, offered slightly greater opportunities to students from the lower economic levels.

Even those professional groups that had started out with a more "lower-class origin"—nursing and pharmacy—attempted to adopt the same procedures as medicine to raise their status. Undoubtedly becoming middle-class is part of the professionalization process, at least in the western world, but it also has implications for medical care that are both positive and negative. Since the time Florence Nightingale established the concept of the "lady" nurse, as distinct from the servant, nursing has been slowly struggling to raise its standards and its status. The hospital schools, the dominant nursing educational institution for the past century, gave students room and board which meant that the financial barriers were kept to a minimum. As collegiate nursing education has grown, and educational standards raised, even hospital schools have turned to charging tuition or fees, and in the process nursing has become less accessible to students from lower socio-economic backgrounds. Pharmacy, which originally had an apprenticeship system, has also become much more middle-class oriented as it transferred into the colleges and the universities.

Regardless of their social-class background, however, once a health professional entered practice, their patients, at least until World War II, were most likely to come from the middle class, and their professional success was dependent upon their ability to attract such patients. This was because medicine, nursing, and dentistry were practiced on a fee-for-service basis in which the relationship between the patient and practitioner was one-to-one. The pharmacist differed from these groups in that he was not usually paid directly for services but for a commodity, his drugs. Nonetheless the implications of such relationships for all health professionals were clear. Even though an individual from a poverty background might have become a professional, his success in monetary terms was dependent upon his ability to escape from his social-class origins.

Outside the system, although not entirely overlooked, were the poor—those unable to pay for the services of an individual practitioner. To deal with these people society established institutions, hospitals, or clinics staffed by medical students, student nurses, interns, or residents who were supervised by a few paid practitioners and several volunteers. At the same time these institutions served as training grounds for the future professional. In effect the poor served as guinea pigs, as we have stated earlier, so that the would-be health professional could acquire enough expertise to deal effectively with the paying patient.

One of the reasons there is a crisis in medicine today is that the institutions originally designed to serve the poor are now also serving the rich. As indicated earlier in this book, the great revolution in medicine of the past 50 years has been the removal of the patient from his home into the hospital, and the change from a one-to-one relationship to the medical team. The change was dictated by several facts, not the least of which was economics. Technical advances in medicine required the purchase of more and more costly equipment and required greater and greater specialization. This meant that services and equipment had to be concentrated and the hospital was the logical place for such concentration. Giving further impetus to this trend was the development of medical insurance, which required hospitalization before reimbursement could be made. This encouraged the transfer to the hospital of many of the services previously carried out in a physician's office or in a patient's home.

The first group to experience the change was nursing; as hospitals grew, nurses changed from being private-duty practitioners to institutional employees. Middle-class patients, forced into the hospital, demanded better care than was available in the student-run charitable institutions. They proved extremely reluctant to be experimented upon by unsupervised nursing and medical students. Hospitals were forced to upgrade their training programs and in doing so they found it much less costly to hire an all-professional nursing staff than to maintain their nursing schools. The change in the nature of the hospitals also coincided with demands of nurses for higher educational standards and as educational requirements were increased nursing became much more middle class. In the process of upgrading itself, nursing delegated many of its functions to new auxiliary nursing personnel: the licensed practical or vocational nurse and the nursing aide who generally came from a lower economic background than the nurse herself.[2]

The transfer of the medical practitioner into the hospital led to a further lengthening of schooling for the physician and the surgeon since the hospital setting required greater and greater specialization. This meant that medical education became even more expensive. Unfortunately, the physician was less able to adjust to the real changes in the nature of medical practice than the nurse, and he often, at least as expressed by the official statements of the American Medical Association, continued to think of medicine as a one-to-one relationship although in reality he was little more than a member of the medical team. Even though he might still be captain of the team, many of his "subordinates" acquired greater expertise in their specialty than he did, and this caused a crisis in the physician's view of himself as well as his subordinates. Dentistry is only now beginning to face up to the same kind of pressures since it has lengthened its period of training and increased its specialization, but the profession is still struggling to avoid team care and is maintaining a one-to-one relationship with the patient. Dentistry still serves the most middle-class clientele of the four groups, since only the middle class can afford this type of health care. The one group which has been downgraded in this process is the pharmacist, who in many ways is overtrained for the tasks demanded of him. The pharmacist is no longer called upon to compound his own prescriptions, but rather to dispense prepared prescription drugs; this means that in most settings he counts pills and measures liquids. He has also lost his place as an individual entrepreneur in the corner drug store as he has become an employee of a chain store.

The middle-class bias so evident in the selection and training of health professionals might well be unconscious; at least it does not appear to be deliberate. The same cannot be said of the professions' handling of either the minority-group patient or the would-be professional from an ethnic minority. Here the exclusion has been conscious and deliberate, and this has had tragic consequences for the health care of Americans.

Discrimination in Medical Education

Until recently medical schools, or at least the vast majority of medical schools, operated on either a discriminatory or a segregated basis. Members of certain minority groups were either trained in segregated institutions or admitted only on quota to a few others. The result of such practices was to keep medicine a much more exclusive profession than it otherwise would have been. Not all segments of the medical community were as segregated or discriminatory as others. Nursing, for example, was somewhat less prone to discriminatory practices than medicine, and within medicine, osteopathic schools were more willing to tolerate minority group members than the others. Inevitably a significant percentage of osteopaths were Jewish, a group which in spite of middle-class origins and aspirations was discriminated against in most orthodox medical schools until the era following World War II. The breakdown of discrimination against Jews in medicine was due in part to a reaction against the ideology of Hitler and a consciousness of what discriminatory attitudes might lead to. Important, also, was a willingness of Jews to organize and support medical schools of their own—such as Einstein College of Medicine or Mount Sinai College of Medicine (now part of the City University of New York)—or to give large-scale financial support to existing schools such as the Chicago College of Medicine. Today it seems that most of the barriers based upon religious identity are in the process of disappearing.

Much more serious barriers, however, were erected against Negroes. As late as 1947 only 20 of the "white" medical schools had Negro students, and then they had only 93 black students in total. There were two segregated medical schools, Howard University Medical School in Washington, D.C., largely funded by the United States Government, and the Meharry Medical College, which is located in Nashville, Tennessee, near Fisk University. This meant that the student who wanted to study medicine and who was Negro had to travel to either of these two centers for his education or wait hopefully for his number on the quota to turn up nearer at home. The effective result was to deny most Negroes the opportunity to become physicians. In 1958, only 2.2 percent of all physicians were Negroes.[3] The percentage has not changed significantly since that time. In 1969, only 2.8 percent of all M.D. candidates were black.[4]

The same discriminatory practices existed in dentistry. Howard University had a dental school, and so did Meharry for a time, but no other dental schools admitted Negroes in any significant number until after World War II. In 1940, for example, there was only one Negro dentist for every 8,745 Negroes compared to the overall ratio of one dentist to 1,865 people.[5] Both Howard University and Meharry Medical College had schools of pharmacy, but most of the other pharmacy schools did not admit Negroes until after World War II.

Nursing also discriminated. In 1950 nonwhite nurses (including Orientals and Indians as well as Negroes) amounted to only 3.5 percent of the total nurse population.[6] Earlier, a study carried out by the American Nurses' Association in 1922 found that only 54 of the accredited nursing schools (there were over 1,000 at the time) admitted Negro students. Twenty-five of these schools were in segregated hospitals maintained by city or county governments, and 19 were in hospitals whose capacity was under 50 beds, then considered the minimum size for a nursing school. Twenty-eight states had no specific school for Negro nurses, which usually meant that there was no opportunity for a Negro nurse to be trained in these states.[7]

By the fall of 1962 there were 1,128 schools of nursing reporting admission policies to the National League for Nursing. Of this number, 22 were predominantly Negro (that is, they had originally been segregated Negro schools) but only nine of them were accredited. Of the remaining schools, 912 said they would accept Negroes as students, 165 would not, and 29 were in the process of closing down. This was some eight years after the 1954 school-desegregating decision. In theory the bulk of the schools were willing to admit Negroes, but indicating a willingness to admit Negroes and actually admitting Negroes often prove to be two different things. In the same year in which the NLN carried out its survey only about 3 percent of the total number of entering students into all associate, baccalaureate, and diploma programs were Negroes.[8] One of the major reasons for this decline was the closing of segregated nursing schools, a procedure which did not immediately lead to an increase in integration in the formerly all-white schools.

Nursing, however, is now showing some improvement. In their most recent survey of minority students the NLN found that in the academic year 1968-1969, 6.2 percent of the students admitted to programs leading to nurse registration were Negro. Still, the percentage that graduated that year was only 3.2 percent, reflecting not only the older admission practices but also the higher drop-out rate of the new minority recruits. Of the various programs for registered nurses, the two-year associate degree programs are the most open, with Negro students comprising 10.5 percent of their total admissions; the baccalaureate programs admitted 6 percent and the diploma programs admitted 3 percent. Negro students are somewhat overrepresented at the practical nurse level, where they comprise 17.4 percent of the total admissions.[9]

It has been only since 1966 that the medical professionals as a group have realized the full effect of their past exclusionary policies on admissions and taken steps not only to say that they were not discriminatory but to recruit minority students. Student demonstrations on many a campus helped emphasize the exclusionary policies of most colleges and universities, and the situation looked much worse in the professional schools. In trying to recruit more minority students, however, the professional schools became conscious of the fact that many of their admission requirements were designed to exclude minorities. Faced with the necessity of turning down the majority of applicants, medical school admission committees have tried to find rational and quantifiable criteria for selection. Though it might be that a kindly disposition is probably as important to the success of a practicing physician as a high grade point average or a high test score, it has been much easier to objectify the grades and tests. Occasionally admission committees, believing that some of the high achievers were better qualified to become research scientists than medical practitioners, went farther down the grade point ladder to admit students, but these efforts were half-hearted and sporadic. Essentially American medical students remained a highly selective intellectual elite, and dental schools make an effective effort to imitate medicine in this regard.

As has been indicated earlier, intellectual achievement at this level is not merely a product of individual genius, it is also a product of social background and schooling. Only a few middle-class minority families could afford to give their children similar advantages and their numbers were not sufficient to satisfy the sudden demand for more identifiable minority students. The ghetto students from segregated schools who made it through the basic baccalaureate training were at a disadvantage when they were thrown in with the student body of a medical school at the graduate level. Those schools which admitted minority students without regard to their educational backgrounds in effect pro-grammed them for failure.[10]

The failure of some of these specially admitted minority students forced a further reexamination of recruitment efforts. It was found that solid compensatory education could give some students the background they needed to compete, and some programs of this type have been started with financing through private foundations or federal grants. The Josiah Macy, Jr. Foundation has been active in this area. Another alternative, however, and one which so far has received little support, is the lowering of the level of medical and dental education for the primary practitioner. As the medical specialties have developed and become more complex, each of them has competed for a place in the basic medical program until medical students are now required to cover each of the various fields far beyond the level needed by the ordinary general practitioner. The Carnegie Founda-tion in a recent study suggested that if medical and dental education were reevaluated, the number of years spent in training could be lessened to three years for the basic medical and dental degrees.[11]

Nursing has been in a somewhat better position to recruit minority students than the more prestigious professions. The entrance requirements for the baccalaureate-level nurse training programs are not so high as those of medicine and dentistry, and the associate degree programs and the hospital training programs are still somewhat lower. In spite of this it was not until deliberate efforts were made that the number of minority students began to increase in any appreciable way. One of the earliest and most successful nursing recruitment programs was that started by the Boston University Alumni in 1965. They called their program ODWIN, an acronym for Opening the Doors Wider in Nursing. Volunteers visited high schools in minority neighborhoods to counsel students and start "future nurse" clubs. With financial assistance from the Rockefeller and Seatlantic funds, they set up tutoring services and programs to provide compensatory education. ODWIN members were not only successful in increasing the number of successful minority students at Boston University but they were able in the succeeding years to spread their program to include other nursing schools in the New England area.[12] The group is now a national membership organization, interested in helping other areas with minority recruitment.

Federal programs have also aided nurse recruitment. For example, the East Los Angeles Health Task Force, financed by the Office of Economic Opportunity (OEO), has a nurse-recruitment project which was started in 1969. It employs three Mexican-American and three black nurse recruiters. Unfortunately, these nurses found that a recruitment program that does not follow-through with scholarship aid and compensatory education can be only partially effective. Although the education gap of many of the underprivileged minority students is not so serious in nursing as it is in medicine or dentistry, segregated education has still left its mark. It would seem that until the education system—or at least that part dealing with the most identifiable minorities—is upgraded, it will be necessary to establish special programs for minority students if we are serious about integrating the health professions.

Negroes, in fact, probably do somewhat better in the health field than some of the other minorities with whom this book is also concerned. Though statistics are difficult to find, it would seem that the percentage of Mexican-Americans, Indians, and Puerto Ricans in the health fields is less than the percentage for Negroes in proportion to their total populations. In recent years, however, Oriental Americans, particularly those with Japanese or Chinese backgrounds, have entered the health fields in greater proportion than their percentage in the population.

Because the past exclusionary policies of American educational institutions have created such a shortage of physicians, the United States has drained neighboring countries of doctors. This is because once an individual has graduated from medical school, even a foreign one, he has comparatively little difficulty in setting up in practice. State licensure often requires special internships, but the obstacles are not so great as to prevent large numbers of physicians from emigrating to the United States. In 1970, for example, it was estimated that one doctor in every 20 trained in Latin America eventually left for the United States.[13] Though few of the Latin American medical schools would meet American standards, they nonetheless supply a large number of American physicians. Many Americans unable to get into medical school in this country go south of the border to one of the Latin American schools that teaches in English to better enable Americans to attend.

Medicine in America has also discriminated against women. A study conducted by Harold I. Kaplan for the National Institute of Mental Health found that in 1970 a significant number of medical schools were still reluctant to accept women as students. Kaplan found that women who were admitted to medical schools were academically more exceptional than their male counterparts. Though women represent about half of the adult population in the United States, only about 7 percent of all physicians are women, compared with 24 percent in Great Britain or 65 percent in the Soviet Union. The major obstacles to the admission of women proved to be, as in the case of other "minorities," the prejudices of the admission committees in medical schools, though these attitudes undoubtedly reflected those of most American medical practitioners.[14] Dentistry is even more closed, as less than 2 percent of the practicing dentists are women.[15] On the other hand, nursing has demonstrated almost as much prejudice toward men, who constituted only 3.5 percent of the registered nurse and 4.4 percent of the practical nurse students in 1969.[16] In the past, hospital schools that required the students to live in dorms on hospital grounds excluded men because they claimed they lacked suitable housing in the nurses' quarters and they were sure interns could not tolerate men nurses in their sections of these buildings. As nursing has entered the colleges and universities, however, it has made little positive effort to recruit men, and this is what is necessary to change long-term patterns.

Discrimination against various minority health practitioners has seriously affected patient care. Obviously a health professional who is white and from the middle class will have trouble communicating with patients who are black and from the lower class. His or her task is made even more difficult if the patient's knowledge of English is less than adequate, as is the case with many Puerto Ricans or Mexican-Americans. Until recently there were Mexican-American patients in Los Angeles County Hospital who were being treated without the benefit of a case history, since neither the nurse nor the physician spoke Spanish; and until pressured to do so, the hospital did not always furnish an interpreter. Much of medical treatment was carried out through sign language.

Patients from different class structures or different ethnic groups than the professional often have difficulty in communicating when both speak the same language. Much of the information we transmit to each other is conveyed by facial expression, body movements, voice tone, and so forth. Professionals who regularly deal with ethnic minorities and who make the effort to understand the subculture can pick up this kind of communication, but most professionals, particularly those who only occasionally deal with the poor of members of minority groups, are totally unaware of their lack of communication.[17] The sex barriers in the health care professions also have implications for patient care because many patients have great difficulty communicating with a professional of the opposite sex. The horror of having to be examined by a male physician keeps many shy Mexican-American women from seeking prenatal care or contraceptive advice. Communication becomes easier as the level of the sophistication of the patient increases, but this does not help the poverty-stricken minority patient.

Discrimination in Treatment

Lack of ability to communicate is only one of the lesser effects of discrimination. A much more serious difficulty, and one which too often has proven fatal to the patient, has been the denial of actual health care to individuals on the basis of race. This aspect of medical discrimination must be counted as one of the most disgraceful chapters in all of American history. In 1954, the year the Supreme Court ordered the desegregation of schools, medical care, both in the North and the South, was delivered on a highly discriminatory basis. A study conducted by the authors of this book in Chicago in that year found that though 15 percent of that city's population (some 590,000 people) were Negro, 50 percent of the Negroes were treated in one hospital, Cook County. This was so in spite of the fact that some of the patients who went there had paid-up hospitalization policies which nominally would have allowed them to be treated at private hospitals. Unfortunately, most of the 65 hospitals in the city, many of which were located in or near the ghetto, refused to admit Negro patients. The results of such discriminatory admission practices were evident in birth statistics. In 1951, 82 percent of the Negro births in Chicago took place in only four hospitals or under the supervision of the Chicago Maternity Center which delivered babies at home. Of the remaining 18 percent of the Negro births, 80 percent were concentrated in eight nongovernmental hospitals. Cook County Hospital alone recorded 54 percent of all Negro births but only 2 percent of the white births.

When a Negro attempted to get treatment at other hospitals, the results were often fatal. We found that a Negro employee of one manufacturing company that had a medical agreement with a hospital was denied admission to the hospital even though he was seriously ill with a massive lobar pneumonia. The hospital admitted Negroes only to "hall" beds which were filled at the time, although there were vacant wards and rooms. More tragically a black journalist from Trinidad who was struck by an automobile and was rushed to a nearby hospital with a skull fracture was denied admission because of his color. After considerable delay he was transferred to Cook County Hospital where he died shortly afterwards. Whether he could have been saved with prompt treatment is perhaps debatable, but a 3-hour delay was certainly fatal.

A 15-year-old Negro boy with an intestinal obstruction was brought by his mother to a private hospital and was denied admission because of his color—despite the woman's ability to pay. He died shortly after arriving at Cook County Hospital. The list of cases compiled in Chicago and elsewhere by the Medical Committee Against Discrimination was full of such incidents.

The extent of discrimination was most effectively revealed when Altgeld Gardens, a public housing project on the far south side of Chicago, contracted with an ambulance service to carry emergency cases past 28 hospitals to Cook County Hospital because of the inability to get treatment any closer. There was an average delay of 1 hour and 20 minutes between the time the ambulance was called and the ambulance arrived at Cook County Hospital. A few of the hospitals on the route did not discriminate, notably Provident Hospital, an all-Negro institution, but it was not equipped to deal with the emergencies from such a large population. In a sense Illinois was a leader among northern states since it had a public accommodation law making it illegal to bar anyone because of race, creed, or color, but hospitals had been ruled as not being "public accommodations."[18] They remained exempt until the legislature amended the state statute in 1955. Still, in 1963 the United States Commission on Civil Rights found medical discrimination in Chicago to be as bad as in Memphis, Tennessee. Most of the Negro patients were still cared for at Cook County Hospital or at three predominantly Negro hospitals, one a proprietary hospital with only 15 beds. Provident Hospital with 206 beds was the largest Negro institution, but the Commission found its facilities outmoded and its treatment for most cases inadequate since its prime purpose was to care for maternity cases.[19]

Compounding the problem was the fact that large numbers of doctors in the United States refused to treat "colored" patients. Even when a physician consented to do so, he could not always gain admission for his patient to a hospital. If he did gain admission for his patient, the patient was usually put into a segregated wing, ward, or hallway, and occasionally in a broom closet. Most Negro physicians lacked hospital affiliations since to have staff or courtesy privileges required membership in the county or state medical society and this in most states was a discriminatory body. To counter such discrimination, Negro physicians early had organized the National Medical Association, which proved over the years to be an effective voice for the Negro physician, but this still did not get him staff privileges.

When students of today hear of such practices their first reaction is to demand that the government do something about it. Unfortunately, in the case of medical discrimination the federal government in the past has tended to encourage rather to discourage such practices. Even after segregation in education had been ruled unconstitutional, the federal government continued to support segregated medical delivery systems and training programs. In fact, it is because so much of the past history of discrimination and segregation has been caused by government intervention that many people now feel it takes positive effort on behalf of the government to undo the damage that it has caused in the past.

One of the most notable examples of governmental encouragement of discriminatory practices was the Hill-Burton Act of 1946, often cited as the Hospital Construction Act. The purpose of the legislation was to provide a government subsidy for the construction of hospitals since a medical census taken at that time found that the number of hospital beds in the United States would have to be doubled to meet the expected demand. Under the legislation the government contributed roughly one-third of the costs incurred in building hospitals in those areas or neighborhoods which met its criteria. Hospital construction immediately zoomed until the three-year period, 1958-1961; hospital construction totaled $1,825,000,000, approximately a third of which came from federal funds.[20]

The Hill-Burton funds, however, provided for hospital construction on a separate-but-equal basis, which meant that very few hospitals were ever constructed for Negroes. By 1963, only 13 new hospitals had been specially constructed for Negroes, while 76 had been specifically designed to exclude Negroes. Inevitably the disparity between white and black medical care increased rather than decreased. In Atlanta, it was found in 1963 that only 630 of the 4,500 hospital beds in the city were available to Negroes—who comprised approximately 50 percent of the population. In Birmingham, Alabama, in that same year, 574 beds were allocated to Negroes and 1,762 to whites—although 40 percent of Birmingham's population was Negro. In some of the smaller southern towns, where only one hospital had been built with Hill-Burton funds, the hospitals refused to admit Negroes under any condition. This was the case in Augusta, Georgia. In fact, Georgia had some 83 hospitals built with grants from the Hill-Burton fund, almost all of which were for whites only.[21]

It was not until 1963, after an estimated 1,000,000 hospital beds had been constructed and over $1,600,000,000 of federal money spent, that the separate-but-equal doctrine in hospital construction finally received a court hearing. In that year six Negro physicians and dentists plus two Negro patients in Greensboro, North Carolina, charged that they were discriminated against by two hospitals, the Moses Cone Memorial Hospital and Wesley Long Community Hospital, both constructed with Hill-Burton aid. The physicians and dentists sought staff or clinic privileges and the two Negro patients sought admission to the hospitals and the right to treatment by their personal physicians. The suit brought by the National Association for the Advancement of Colored People also received support from the Department of Justice. After an adverse decision in the local court, the Fourth Circuit Court of Appeals in Richmond, Virginia, struck down the separate-but-equal clause as unconstitutional and this decision was affirmed by the United States Supreme Court.[22]

The decision, known in the law books as *Simkins* vs. *Moses H. Cone Memorial Hospital,* forced the government to change its policy from that of promoting segregation to that of being an advocate of nondiscrimination. The Public Health Service, then charged with administering the Hill-Burton funds, eventually passed regulations prohibiting discrimination by any hospital which in the future received construction funds. More positive action came in 1964 with the passage of the Civil Rights Act. Title VI of that act carried a prohibition against the denial of benefits under any program or activity receiving federal financial assistance on grounds of race, color, or national origin. Each federal department or agency extending financial assistance, other than by contract of insurance or guarantee, was directed to effectuate this prohibition by rules approved by the President and authorized to terminate assistance to those agencies which failed to comply. In spite of Title VI, most hospitals which had discriminated in the past (including those previously built with Hill-Burton funds) continued to do so since reimbursements for patients usually came third-hand, from local welfare agencies, and the state agencies which managed the federal funds were reluctant to enforce the prohibitions against discrimination. In a survey made by the United States Commission on Civil Rights one year after the passage of the act, medical discrimination was found to be widespread. Negroes were housed in segregated wings or floors, forced to use separate waiting rooms, nurseries, cafeterias and clinics, and in many cases Negroes were entirely excluded from the medical facilities. Negro physicians were refused staff privileges at any but all-Negro or inner-city hospitals. Most nursing homes were restricted to whites, although a large percentage of the patients were supported by federally assisted public welfare agencies. Those nursing homes admitting Negroes were usually all-black institutions. Even state owned or operated health facilities, such as mental health institutions, tuberculosis sanitariums, and charity hospitals, were often segregated by state law.[23]

The most effective instrument in encouraging a change in past practices was the enactment of Medicare on July 3, 1965, since in line with Title VI all participating hospitals and nursing homes, public or private, had to drop their discriminatory practices in order to qualify for funds. This was emphasized in 1966 by a White House directive which stated that no hospital that discriminated would be eligible for Medicare funds. To make certain the directive was enforced, the Office of Equal Health Opportunity (OEHO) was established in the Public Health Service in February 1966 to screen hospitals applying for Medicare funds to see that they did not discriminate. In July 1966, when Medicare became effective, OEHO reported that more than three thousand hospitals which in the past had used discriminatory assignments or had segregated facilities had agreed to integrate. This was one-third of the 9,200 hospitals in the United States at that time. By 1968 it was estimated that over 98 percent of the hospitals applying for Medicare met the nondiscriminatory provisions of the Civil Rights Act.

Regarded as typical of the changes taking place was the example of St. Dominic Jackson Memorial Hospital in Jackson, Mississippi. Before 1963 no Negro doctors had been allowed staff privileges at the hospital, no Negro students had been accepted into the nursing training program, and all Negro patients had been confined to a first-floor ward. Negro newborns, however, had been kept in a segregated section of the nursery on the second floor. In 1965 the hospital admitted Negroes to its nursing school and granted staff privileges to a few Negro physicians. Shortly afterwards, Negro fathers were allowed to visit the second floor to see their babies in the nursery, a privilege previously denied them. Still, by 1968 the hospital had little biracial occupancy. In order to speed up integration the OEHO took legal action in cities such as Pittsburgh, Baltimore, and Camden (New Jersey) to break down entrenched patterns of staff privileges and patient referrals.[24]

In extreme cases, the government acted to cut off funds. An early test case involved the Alabama Board of Mental Health which administered Bryce, Searcy, and Partlow Hospitals. At Bryce, Negro and white patients were housed in different buildings and no Negro professional staff members were employed although Negro psychiatric aides were assigned to Negro wards. The treatment center, an adjunct to Bryce Hospital, admitted only Negro patients and provided inferior services and facilities. Searcy Hospital was an all-Negro hospital with inferior facilities. Partlow Hospital assigned patients to wards on a racial basis, segregating psychiatric aides' dining rooms and assigning them patients only of their own race. Because of such practices a hearing officer ordered termination of all federal funds on October 4, 1967. In spite of objections from the hospital, the hearing officer was upheld.

Though this might be interpreted as a forward step, the difficulty in carrying integration much beyond tokenism is indicated by the case of the Mobile Infirmary, the largest hospital in Alabama but the one which has the fewest Negroes. In 1966 it was found that only 20 of the 1,767 patients admitted during a one-month period were Negro. The application of the infirmary for Medicare funds was deferred for three months while an investigation was carried out, but the infirmary successfully argued that it was in compliance with Title VI since few Negroes chose to go there. Though it was assumed that there was an active policy of discouraging Negroes, and it was evident that Negroes feared the treatment they would receive if they did attend the clinic, the OEHO ruled that it could find no Negroes who claimed to have been denied admission.[25]

If government efforts to integrate hospitals have not been particularly vigorously carried through, they have done little or nothing to integrate nursing homes or to make more space available to Negroes. This situation exists in spite of the fact that the federal government has been dispensing at least a quarter of a billion dollars annualy to nursing homes to care for elderly patients. OEHO did circulate questionnaires about discriminatory practices, and all nursing homes receiving federal funds signed assurances of nondiscrimination, but no effective enforcement or supervision has been carried out as of this writing.

Concluding Comments

Obviously one of the major factors working against better health care in the United States has been the past discriminatory practices of medical institutions and medical practitioners. In spite of recent government effort, medical practice is still discriminatory and often segregated. There is also still a double standard for medical treatment in the country, as poor people still receive second-rate medical care from practitioners who have little understanding of their problems. Though the federal government after years of giving tacit support to discrimination and segregation finally started to take some positive steps in 1964 to eliminate these evils, years of accumulated practices and attitudes cannot so easily be overcome. Our health care delivery system remains uneven and until there are changes the United States will still continue to lag behind other countries in the health of its citizens.

Notes

1. Herman M. Somer and Anne R. Somer, *Doctors, Patients and Health Insurance: The Organization and Financing of Medical Care* (Washington, D.C.: The Brookings Institution, 1961).
2. Vern and Bonnie Bullough, *The Emergence of Modern Nursing,* 2nd ed. (New York: Macmillan, 1969).
3. Dietrich C. Reitzes, *Negroes and Medicine* (Commonwealth Fund Study published by Harvard University Press, Cambridge, Mass., 1958), pp. xxi and xxii.
4. The Carnegie Commission on Higher Education, *Higher Education and the Nation's Health: Policies for Medical and Dental Education* (New York: McGraw-Hill, 1970), p. 28.
5. Clifton Orrin Dummett, *The Growth and Development of the Negro in Dentistry* (Chicago: The Stanek Press for the National Dental Association, 1952).
6. American Nurses' Association, *Facts About Nursing* (New York: ANA, 1958), p. 10.
7. *Nursing Outlook* (February 1965), p. 63, a boxed extract from *The Trained Nurse and Hospital Review* 74 (March 1925), p. 260.
8. M. Elizabeth Carnegie, "Are Negro Schools of Nursing Needed Today?" *Nursing Outlook* 12 (February 1964), pp. 52-56, reprinted in *New Directions for Nurses,* edited by Bonnie and Vern Bullough (New York: Springer, 1971), pp. 292-303.

9. "Educational Preparation for Nursing—1969" *Nursing Outlook* 18 (September 1970), pp. 52-57.
10. Julian C. Stanley, "Predicting College Success of the Educationally Disadvantaged," *Science* 171 (February 1971), pp. 640-646.
11. The Carnegie Commission on Higher Education, *op. cit.*, pp. 35-59.
12. Jean Scheinfeldt, "Opening Doors Wider in Nursing," *American Journal of Nursing* 67 (July 1967), pp. 1461-1464.
13. Francis B. Kent, "Latin America Losing Much Needed Doctors," *Los Angeles Times*, September 17, 1971.
14. A summary of this report was written by Elizabeth Shelton, "Prejudices Hit Women in Medicine," *Los Angeles Times*, October 4, 1970.
15. The Carnegie Commission on Higher Education, *op. cit.*, p. 26.
16. "Educational Preparation for Nursing—1969", *op. cit.*
17. For a brief article on this topic see Gloria D. Bigham, "To Communicate with Negro Patients," *American Journal of Nursing* 64 (September 1964), pp. 113-115.
18. The information was collected together in a pamphlet by Bonnie and Vern Bullough and Leo Tannenbaum, *What Color Are Your Germs?* (Chicago Committee To End Medical Discrimination, 1954).
19. U.S. Commission on Civil Rights, *Civil Rights '63* (Washington, D.C.: U.S. Government Printing Office, 1963), pp. 137-138.
20. Seymour E. Harris, *The Economics of American Medicine* (New York: Macmillan, 1964), p. 170.
21. U.S. Commission on Civil Rights, *op. cit.*, p. 131.
22. Max Seham, "Discrimination Against Negroes in Hospitals," *New England Journal of Medicine*, 271 (October 29, 1964), pp. 940-943.
23. 323 F. 2d 939 (4th Cir)., cert. denied, 376 U.S. 938 (1964). See also Max Seham, *op. cit.*
24. See the U.S. Commission on Civil Rights, *Title VI Circuit One Year After: A Survey of Desegregation of Health and Welfare Services in the South* (Washington, D.C.: U.S. Government Printing Office, 1966). See also "The Impact of Title VI on Health Facilities," *The George Washington Law Review* 36 (May 1968), pp. 980-993.
25. "The Impact of Title VI on Health Facilities," *op. cit.*

9

Improving Health Care Delivery

Today's world is radically changed from that of the past, yet American medicine, in spite of its tremendous advances, often seems to act as if the United States were still primarily a nation of small towns and rural farms. Over the past century millions of people have moved from the country to the large urban complexes until today, less than 5 percent of the population is engaged in agriculture. In the rural environment, a man, within limits, could be self-reliant, making his own clothes, growing his own crops, and when calamity threatened, his neighbors or family were usually there to help. Medically he could learn to know and love a physician who, in a time of crisis, often spent long hours with him. If it was necessary to hire a nurse she came to the patient's home and cared for him on a one-to-one basis.

In the city, on the other hand, almost everything a person does is dependent upon the impersonal activities of large numbers of other people as the city is preeminently the home of the specialist. Such a simple task as getting to work takes the coordinated efforts of dozens of people whether one takes a subway, a bus, or drives his own car. In health care, the individual has been replaced by a team of specialists who individually often do not know what the others are doing. At best, the system is often confusing, and all too frequently it breaks down. An example of the difficulties was outlined by Dr. Milton Roemer, Professor of Public Health at UCLA, in his testimony before the Senate Subcommittee on the Health of the Elderly in 1967.

> May I take the time of a distinguished committee of the U.S. Senate to tell of one aged patient who, like most old people, suffered from multiple diagnoses?
>
> He had a serious eye problem—actually two diseases: glaucoma and keratitis—for which he received care at a nearby medical center, in the department of ophthalmology.
>
> His personal doctor, a good internist, however, had diagnosed a mild diabetes and for this periodic visits were necessary to an office eight miles away.
>
> Painful corns and bunions, impairing the ability to walk, were not within the specialty of the personal doctor, so these required periodic visits to a podiatrist at an office six miles in another direction.
>
> Dental care, in an effort to save the few remaining teeth, so that dentures would fit more firmly and food could be more properly chewed required numerous visits to a dentist at still another location.
>
> Then a bladder problem developed and prostatic disease was suspected. At about the same period, the patient showed lethargy and confusion, suggesting a mild cerebrovascular accident. The personal doctor made a home call and the decision was to hospitalize.
>
> A bed was not immediately available—except in a small proprietary hospital which the family refused—and it was not till ten days later that he could be admitted to a good voluntary general hospital fifteen miles away.
>
> After x-rays, cystoscopy, and other examinations there, his treatment was stabilized. In the workup, it was discovered that a drug the ophthalmologist had been prescribing for many months was causing serious side effects which had been missed by the internist since these two specialists had never communicated with each other.
>
> The patient was then admitted to a sanitarium selected for its closeness to the family home, so that visits from the patient's children would be possible daily.
>
> This was one of the 'better' nursing homes—it was certainly expensive enough at $32 a day paid by Medicare—but this was evidently not costly enough to support a proper staff. After a few days, because of lack of proper surveillance, this aged patient was found roaming on the street. When this happened a second time,

*the commercial proprietor decided to discharge the patient as
'too difficult to care for.' It took five weeks of nursing care at
home, with daily problems of incontinence of urine and feces,
before a bed in another nursing home became available.*

*The later facility proved to be better managed and the
patient improved. After only two weeks, however, he was getting
up from a chair one day when he fell and fractured his left hip.*

*This required an orthopedic surgeon, readmission to the
hospital, and preparation for a major operation. But then
complications to the diabetes set in, because of the traumatic
shock of the fracture. A delay in over twenty-four hours in
reporting a critical laboratory test nearly cost the patient's life at
this time. Had the hospital been adequately staffed, this delay
would not have occurred.*

*A skillful operation, with a pinning of the broken bone was
done. Special-duty nurses costing $111 a day—over and above the
Medicare coverage of the hospital bill—had to be hired because of
the shortage of regular hospital nurses.*

*I have not recounted the other details of multiple drug
prescriptions, special services of an appliance shop to adjust the
bed at home, the physical therapy required for a knee injury, and
much more.*[1]

Dr. Roemer added that the patient in question was his widowed
father who had retired after fifty-one years of medical practice. If
Dr. Roemer, with his medical background and knowledge, found it
difficult to wend his way through the maze of specialists in
securing adequate medical care, it should be evident that those
with much less ability to deal with the medical establishment
would have even greater difficulties. Urbanization with its great
potential for specialization has encouraged a jungle of specialists
and an impossible medical care delivery system.

Tied in with urbanization has been the growth of technology, which has made human labor less important as machines
have taken over more of the functions once reserved for brains and
muscles. This has meant that many types of work have been
upgraded so that the average worker now has to have more skills
or be better educated than he did in the past. In the case of
medicine this trend has led to a proliferation of devices and
techniques, higher educational standards, and greater gaps between
the various levels of health practitioners. Not too long ago most
medical care was in the hands of a physician, a nurse, or a
pharmacist, but now there are some 35 major categories of jobs

within the health care industry which in terms of total manpower is the third largest industry in the United States and one of the most rapidly growing segments of the economy.

Together technology and urbanization have tended to widen the gap between the "haves" and "have nots" in all societies. In the United States many of the "have nots" are members of groups which traditionally have been discriminated against in American life, and their immediate situation is likely to worsen before it improves. In fact, the hardest hit by the changing employment standards have been the undereducated, particularly members of minority groups, who, in spite of the civil rights legislation of the last two decades, often find themselves still at a disadvantage because of past economic and educational discrimination.

This means that health care, more than ever before, is inevitably tied in with the economic conditions of mass numbers of people. Over the past century Americans have taken steps to lessen the economic extremes through the enactment of a graduated income tax, the inauguration of a system of social security, and the establishment of various kinds of government-supported welfare programs. Medically we have enacted Medicare and Medicaid as supplements to Social Security, as well as various smaller-scale programs aimed at certain groups of people or specific disease entities. However, most health care is still privately paid for on a fee-for-service or insurance basis. This means that people who do not have money to buy good health care are not likely to get it. Nearly 200 years ago Thomas Malthus, an English clergyman, wrote *An Essay on the Principle of Population* in which he said:

> *I believe it has been generally remarked by those who have attended to bills of mortality that of the number of children who die annually, much too great a proportion belongs to those who may be supposed unable to give their offspring proper food and attention, exposed as they are occasionally to severe distress and confined, perhaps to unwholesome habitations and hard labor.*

In 1966 Alonzo Yerby could quote Malthus as summarizing contemporary conditions in America and describe the medical care of the poor as piecemeal, poorly organized, and without compassion or concern for the dignity of the individual.[2]

The Gordian Knot

There are no easy answers to our current health deficiencies. Problems are intertwined and interrelated until there is almost a Gordian knot, impossible to unravel except as Alexander the Great did—by cutting it with a sword and starting over. Although we are not advocating a revolution, it does seem obvious that a drastic revision of the health care delivery system is needed to replace the present complex, patchwork nonsystem with a comprehensive and accessible plan for the delivery of health care to all of the people. However, even with a rational system of health care there will still be inequities in health until problems of discrimination and poverty are solved.

As was indicated in the previous chapter, a concentrated effort to eliminate the barriers due to segregation and discrimination in health care institutions is still needed. The schools which prepare health professionals should open their doors in meaningful ways so that members of minority groups can be better represented in the ranks of their graduates, and health workers at all levels need to examine their own attitudes towards poor and minority patients. There are probably enough laws on the books to deal with these types of discrimination, but existing laws need better enforcement both at the overt level and on the more subtle personal level.

This book is not the place to go into the whole strategy of ending poverty since our primary emphasis is on health, but health itself, as it has been emphasized before, is dependent on ending poverty. The complexity of dealing with poverty makes us cautious in proposing any one solution. Many investigators advocate a Guaranteed Annual Wage as a means of fighting poverty, others the development of WPA-like projects to provide jobs, others a cut in working hours, and still others a vast overhaul of the welfare system.

Robert Heilbroner has argued that a good measure of a country's greatness is the way in which it treats its sick, its poor, and its deviants. If such a measure is applied on a world basis it becomes obvious that the United States, in spite of its great power and strength, is overshadowed by large numbers of nations in the world. Heilbroner believes that our relative failure in this regard is due to an American antiwelfare animus, a feeling that those who do not succeed have no one to blame but themselves. This attitude has led to an anesthetizing of America's social conscience that, coupled with a profound suspicion of government, has caused us to regard poverty with mixed feelings of indifference and impotence.[3] If Heilbroner is right, and Americans are indifferent to social neglect and reluctant to use public authority to deal with it, then health care will continue to be in a crisis and poverty will grow. In an earlier and more rural day, personal charity could help ease the burdens, but in this day of urban problems government action becomes imperative, and fortunately or unfortunately even local governments are no longer able to deal with it. In the past when government has entered into the poverty area it has mostly been through the city or county, less often through the state, and only rarely through agencies of the federal government itself. The result has been a patchwork of welfare programs which varies from state to state and even locality to locality, with the greatest crisis in the largest urban areas—the political unit least able to deal with the problem because of the present tax structure and distribution of political power. In order to work effectively toward a solution, we have to recognize that poverty and health care are national problems.[4]

There are still approximately 25.5 million persons in the United States who fall below the poverty lines. Between 1959 to 1969 the number classified at the poverty level had been declining, but in that year it once again began to increase and has continued to do so.[5] In part the change represented a change in attitudes of administrations from President Johnson to President Nixon, but it has also been a result of the continuing on-going technological revolution. The most severe contraction in the job market has been at the unskilled level, which means that the unemployment has fallen heaviest on the least educated segment of society. Since most of these workers traditionally have lacked the union organization or professional associations of the more sophisticated workers, they have no organized advocates for their position. If poverty is associated with unemployment, and to a large degree it is, then the obvious answer is more employment, but this apparently is much easier said than done.

The most concentrated recent effort to eliminate poverty was made by President Lyndon B. Johnson in 1964 when he declared a "war on poverty." The opening battle in his war was the passage of the Economic Opportunity Act, which recognized that one of the problems of the long-term or chronically unemployed was a lack of faith in themselves, an alienation from the system. To overcome this the EOA attempted to encourage "maximum feasible participation" of the poverty population in solving their own problems. Grants were given to local groups who were willing to try innovative or grass-roots approaches to solving problems related to poverty. The result was a variety of programs including occupational training, health clinics, neighborhood services, and Head Start nursery schools. Unfortunately the escalation of the Vietnam war tended to take public attention and government resources away from the war on poverty and President Nixon decided to phase out most of the EOA programs.

In his critique of the war on poverty, Daniel Patrick Moynihan, who served as an advisor to Presidents Johnson and Nixon, held that the program had been contaminated from the start by too close a relationship to sociologists who held that the alienation of the poverty population was a basic cause of the continued cycle of poverty. This orientation, Moynihan believed, led to the attempt to get the active participation of the poor and in his opinion caused its failure.[6] His criticism cannot be dismissed lightly but it still does not answer the problem of how to overcome alienation. From our point of view the failure lies more in the somewhat naive expectation that alienation could be ended overnight rather than in the recognition of its existence. While it is true that, instead of the poor, the major participants in planning often came to be politicians, social workers, revolutionaries, and even a few opportunists, a surprising number of the genuinely poor became motivated. Unfortunately for public opinion, strife followed as the various groups fought for control of the local poverty money.

Probably a more basic difficulty with the program was that it depended on grants to local agencies to finance programs which supposedly would prove their worth and then be picked up by state and local governments or private agencies. These assumptions were simply erroneous. Few state or local governments had the interest or money to pick up on programs, and most private agencies had their hands full with the tasks they were already doing. The dependence on grants also created administrative problems. In theory the grant system avoids a large bureaucracy and allows for greater individual initiative. In practice, however, innovation depends not only upon those who are applying for grants but also upon those who award them. Since the grants were awarded by a bureaucracy, innovation was limited to what the bureaucracy was willing to fund. To their credit they often looked with favor upon innovative programs, but not always. Moreover, the Office of Economic Opportunity programs as a whole were wasteful of both time and money. Much of the time, energy, and talent of local OEO officials and the staffs of participating agencies were spent in writing grant proposals. Once funded, much of the actual money went into administrative overhead instead of directly into the project. Still, when all such criticisms have been made, there was a surprising amount of success and many of the programs proved their effectiveness. In the health field one of the most successful OEO programs was the training and employment of home health aides and social work assistants whose origins were in the community being served. In part, such programs were successful because they did the obvious, they offered jobs to the unemployed, but agencies also found that these new employees were extremely valuable because of their ability to understand and interpret both the clients' and agency's point of view.[7]

The OEO demonstration health centers—such as the two clinics opened by the Tufts University School of Medicine in the Columbia Point housing project in Massachusetts and in Mound Bayou, Mississippi, or the Multipurpose Health Center in Watts—have been successful in demonstrating that it is possible to give comprehensive health care and that members of the poverty community can be involved in planning and in giving health care.[8] However, such successful projects serve to emphasize that scattered, token clinics, which give care only to residents of a specified geographical area, are not enough. In fact, they serve as stark reminders that comprehensive care is not available to all poor Americans.

Health Care Delivery System

This country desperately needs to replace its patchwork nonsystem for financing health care with a comprehensive, federally run system of national health insurance. For many years now the United States has been the only industrialized country which does not have some kind of national health insurance or national health service.[9] Usually the failure to develop such a system is blamed on the American Medical Association, and although this is a much too simplistic explanation, the AMA has certainly been a significant force in "saving us from socialized medicine." For a long time the organization was in the hands of general practitioners who were fighting against the increasing specialization of medicine. In part the doctors who were most active in organizational activities were also likely to come from smaller towns, so that in a sense, the 20th-century struggle within the AMA represented an alliance of the small towns against the big cities, of rural versus urban, and of old American values against the new. Over the years, while the ultraconservative forces held sway, the organization fought against private health insurance, maternal health programs, various aspects of the social security legislation, medical care for military dependents, and even against Veterans Administration hospitals.[10]

The AMA is still a conservative organization—in part because the very nature of medical practice tends to leave the average doctor with little time for organizational activities. This means that the association is usually dominated by the older retired physicians who are still thinking both politically and medically in terms of their own youth. Too often they assume that medical care is still given on a one-to-one basis with a fee for service. While physicians have generally been noted for their compassion, the heavily science-oriented focus of medical education has given them little background with which to understand the problems of the modern world, and their too-heavy work schedule has left them little time for independent study.

Although the attitudes and actions of the AMA still affect the way in which the medical establishment works today, as will be indicated later, no lobby—and the AMA is a lobby—can be effective unless it expresses the views of a large segment of its members as well as the general population. For a long time the AMA attitudes were the dominant American ones, but increasingly nurses, hospital administrators, public health officials, and others have broken with the AMA while the balance of power within that organization has shifted somewhat to the urban practitioner. The result has been a modification of some of the earlier political positions. There is also a growing number of doctors, usually young ones, who have refused to join the organization. Some of these rebels have joined with other health workers to form dissident groups such as the Medical Committee for Human Rights or Physicians for Social Responsibility, but large numbers of others remain unorganized as the salaried medical positions have helped weaken the power of the AMA because they cannot use denial of hospital positions as a negative sanction to force membership.

Other Countries

Germany under Prince Otto von Bismarck was the first country in the world to establish a compulsory national sickness insurance program. The original program, started in 1883, gave free care only to enrolled workers but benefits were soon extended to the families of employed persons. Following the German example, several other European countries took steps to have their government enter into the medical field—including Austria in 1888, Sweden in 1891, Denmark in 1892, Belgium in 1894, and Switzerland in 1912. England acted much more slowly and in a more piecemeal fashion. Some compensation was given to a few workers in 1880, and a limited national health insurance program was enacted in 1911, but complete health coverage was not established until the inauguration of National Health Insurance in 1948. The Union of Soviet Socialist Republics nationalized all health care in 1917 as part of the Russian Revolution, and other countries which came under the Russian sphere of influence following World War II patterned their health care delivery system after that of the Russians. There are numerous other countries which have also adopted some form of government-sponsored or controlled health care.

In spite of the fact that the various government-sponsored plans are usually labeled "socialized medicine" by the AMA and its supporters, there is a vast difference in the way each country administers its programs: some are based on a fee for service, some on cash reimbursement, others on a capitation basis, others on straight salaries. Each system has its advantages and disadvantages. The difficulty with the negotiated or set fee-for-service system is that the better-paid procedures tend to be more frequently performed than those paid less because the physician is likely to opt for the more expensive treatment than the lower-cost one. Moreover, failure to pay adequately for certain procedures can result in the underdevelopment of an entire speciality. Fee-for-service benefits the surgical specialties more than the medical or preventive specialties since the surgical specialties can easily be itemized and priced. In those systems in which any doctor can be paid for any procedure, general practitioners become more alike in skills and income, and specialists become more versatile since the narrower the specialization the more difficult it is to establish a set fee. Fee-for-service systems also enable the physician to bill the funds without the patient's knowledge since there is little witness to the actual work as against the physician's claims. Under this system it is possible to write fee schedules with variable payment formulas that discourage the unnecessary multiplication of work, but the problem is to prevent these formulas from discouraging justified long-term care.[11]

An example of a country where fee-for-service is practiced is Germany. Originally the German system arranged for individuals to join a sickness fund and this fund then contracted for care from groups of doctors. At the present time there are about 200 such funds in operation in West Germany, covering about 87 percent of the population. Within the group the patients can choose their own general practitioner but are referred to specialists only as needed. Physicians are paid on the basis of a fee-for-service with fee levels being negotiated by the sickness funds and the local association of doctors. Hospitals are run by local government and their staffs, physicians as well as nurses, are salaried. Although satisfaction with the system is high, some 90 percent of those enrolled recently indicated they would remain if it were voluntary instead of compulsory, it is not without problems. In order to get reimbursement, physicians with few patients tend to require more visits per patient than the busy physicians. In a 1966 study it was found that doctors who saw 2,500 to 3,000 patients per calendar quarter provided 5.06 services per person while those seeing 1,000 to 1,500 provided 6.24 services and those seeing fewer than 1,000 provided 8.90. From this it would seem that at least some of those extra visits to the practitioner with the small patient load may have been motivated by a desire to keep up income. From the physician members the greatest complaint is the amount of paperwork required to gain reimbursement. From the governmental point of view the system is expensive to operate unless there is very rigid fee control.[12]

Closely allied to the negotiated fee-for-service system, but with more difficulties and complications in operation, is the cash benefit system. Instead of receiving a fee for his service, the physician charges cash and then the patient is reimbursed. This system has the advantage of being the most politically feasible in those countries where there are well-established medical practitioners—such as in the United States. The physicians are usually more willing to accept this reimbursement procedure because they believe that it will preserve their autonomy in full because the patient, not the physician, communicates with the sick fund. When this system has been tried these beliefs as expressed by the medical profession have been proven wrong because physicians who charge higher rates for the same service soon find themselves being queried by the reimbursement agency and those who persist find themselves under investigation. Inevitably many doctors are placed under sanctions by the government, even to the point that patients going to them are not reimbursed. Most cash benefit systems also anticipate that the patient will pay part of the initial charge, but the effect of this is to discourage the poor from ever seeking needed medical care or waiting until an emergency arises. In order to get around this it has become necessary to impose means tests, the very thing that national health insurance was supposed to eliminate. The cash payment system also has most of the other difficulties of fee for service. Nevertheless, both France and Sweden have established cash benefit systems which from the doctor's point of view have the advantage of giving high incomes to the doctor. Both countries have also achieved better results in medical care for the poor than the United States.[13]

Capitation as it is operated in England is much simpler to administer than fee-for-service or cash benefit systems, but it also has difficulties. Under the English system a doctor is responsible for a panel of patients, which means that the quality of his service is dependent upon his own conscience or the informal sanctions of other members of the profession. At worst, the system gives little encouragement for the physician to do more than the minimum required for the patient, but it also discourages unnecessary or drastic medical procedures. If a physician has a time-consuming patient he might want to transfer him to another panel or to an outpatient department of a hospital unless there are effective administrative or ethical deterrents for him not to do so. The English system also reinforces a distinction between the general practitioner and the specialist by depriving the general practitioner of any financial motive to perform tasks assigned to the specialist. It has the merit, from the physician's point of view, of preserving the individual practitioner in his office, and in England and Holland, where the capitation system is most firmly established, general practitioners were traditionally based in private offices, separate from the specialists who were attached to the hospitals.[14]

The English system has the advantage of offering almost universal coverage. Each patient is assigned to a panel, and there are similar panels for dental care and drugs. Specialists and hospital employees are on a direct salary under the direction of the Ministry of Health. The chief dissatisfaction with the capitation system comes not from patients, but from physicians. Many physicians feel their pay is low and to increase it they take on rather large patient panels, an average of 2,300 patients. To handle so many patients, they then have to work long hours and cannot spend as much time with each patient as careful medical practice would indicate is desirable. The separation of the general practitioner from the patient in the hospital and lack of contact with specialists also reduces the intellectual stimulation of seeing the seriously ill patient or working with colleagues. This is not so much a difficulty with capitation per se, but with the way health care delivery is organized in England.[15]

Most countries that have national health schemes rely heavily upon salaried physicians, although even here there is great variance in medical care because the delivery system seems to be dependent on past tradition within the country. In many ways the salary system encourages desirable characteristics such as non-mercenary attitudes, close colleague relationships, interest in personal professional growth, and it also has the virtue of greater administration simplicity than the other systems. The salaried system also discourages unnecessary treatment or medically unjustified multiplication of procedures, although in the few systems in which doctors earn overtime or can select the amount of salaried work time, this is a problem. Under a salary system, also, medical care can be more equitably distributed through encouraging medical practitioners to go into areas of greatest need by giving them higher salaries to do so. In salaried systems which also allow the physician to have a private practice the more affluent patients are often referred to the individual doctor in his private practice hours, thus subverting the system somewhat. This is particularly true in countries like Egypt where salaries for physicians are low.[16]

Russia and most of those countries which have followed the Russian lead have adopted the salary system. In Russia all levels of health workers are salaried, and care is given through a system of polyclinics, health centers, and hospitals. In line with earlier Russian tradition there is considerable opportunity for advancement within the system and theoretically a hospital orderly or an ambulance driver can work his way up through a system of additional training programs to become a physician. In actuality this sort of upward mobility is uncommon although nurses and feldshers, the middle-level medical workers, occasionally move up the career ladder to become physicians. Soviet doctors give fewer diagnostic tests and treatments than do Western physicians but this may be due less to salary than to a clinical tradition which for a long time suffered from a shortage of equipment, technicians, and laboratories. The Soviet system of medicine is one of the most popular governmental services in the USSR, and even the personnel shortages and time pressures of World War II did not lead to dissatisfaction. The Harvard Russian Research Center, for example, interviewed Russian émigres shortly after the war and found a remarkably high level of satisfaction with the doctor-patient relationship. Those refugees who eventually settled in America felt that one of the few advantages

Russia had over the American system was in their medical care delivery system.[1][7]

There are other variations of payment for health care delivery, and in fact many countries have combinations of several, as does the United States today. All of the systems, however, at least in the industrialized nations, tend to offer adequate medical care and have the advantage of reaching segments of the population not reached by the American system. This does not mean that the United States should adopt any of the systems per se—in part because American medicine has a different tradition— but that there are many kinds of variations possible even in "socialized" medicine.

The Struggle for Health Insurance in the United States

The attempt to gain a national health insurance in this country has been, and continues to be, a long and bitter struggle. In the process of the struggle American medicine has developed along certain lines which have to be considered in planning a better health care delivery system. In order to understand the importance of this early struggle in forming medical practice today it is necessary to examine some of the past history of medical insurance, if only briefly. One of the early leaders in the campaign for government-sponsored health insurance was Dr. Alexander Lambert, an AMA leader, who was also personal physician to President Theodore Roosevelt. He had enough influence to get compulsory health insurance included in the platform of the Progressive Party platform in 1912 when Theodore Roosevelt attempted to regain the presidency. It was several decades, however, before the Democratic or Republican parties picked up this part of the Bull Moose or Progressive party platform. With the failure of the Roosevelt campaign, much of the early efforts to gain some sort of health service was directed by a private reform group called the American Association for Labor Legislation, which had originally been established to lobby for workmen's compensation laws in various states. As this movement succeeded (some 41 states had enacted laws by 1920) the association turned its attention to the health problems. In its early attempt to establish health insurance the AALL for a brief time had the support of the AMA, which between 1915 to 1920 was at its progressive best under the influence and leadership of Lambert, I. M. Rubinow, and others who were members of an AMA Social Insurance Committee established in 1915. By 1920, however, in part due to grass-roots opposition by doctors, the AMA had adopted a policy of official opposition to any kind of health insurance, private or public.

The model health insurance bill drawn up by AALL providing for broad hospital and medical coverage to workers and their families on a state level was introduced into 20 state legislatures between 1914 and 1920, and some nine states appointed special commissions to deal with the subject. None of the bills passed and the movement almost died during the 1920s. Employers were generally antagonistic on the ground that their costs would be increased. Commercial life insurance companies became active opponents, even though at that time they wrote little health insurance. The AALL plan, however, included a funeral benefit which the insurance companies opposed and they also had in effect about six billion dollars of industrial insurance. Even organized labor, particularly in the person of Samuel Gompers, president of the AFL, opposed the health scheme on the grounds that it would lead to government control of the union movement. Many state federations, however, were in favor, and it was the state labor organizations which gave the greatest support to the effort. Large pharmaceutical houses also opposed the various bills as did an increasing number of local medical societies and individual doctors whose opposition eventually led the AMA itself to oppose the plan. In California, where the state consti-tution permitted a referendum, an attempt to set up a state-sponsored health insurance plan was overwhelmingly defeated at the polls.[18]

The issue was not dead, only dormant. Continuing concern over the cost and organization of medical care by 1925 had resulted in a Washington Conference on the Economic Factors Affecting the Organization of Medicine. A second conference was held in 1926 and this led in 1927 to the formation of a Committee on the Costs of Medical Care under the chairmanship of Ray Lyman Wilbur, Secretary of the Interior. For the next five years the Committee, with the support of various private foundations, investigated the costs of medical care. Its findings and recommendations filled some 28 volumes, and there were a number of subsidiary reports in addition. The final summary, entitled *Medical Care for the American People*, appeared in 1932 when the country was at the depth of the depression.[19] It included both a majority and a minority report. The majority favored medical and hospital insurance on a voluntary basis until adequate experience could be accumulated to serve as a sound basis for a comprehensive system based upon compulsory tax deductions. The majority also approved group medical practice organized around health centers, and grants-in-aid to provide hospitals, doctors, and nurses to poor and thinly populated areas. It also urged government support of the cost of medical care for the indigent, the tubercular, and the mentally ill. The minority, on the other hand, opposed any kind of prepaid medical care even on a voluntary basis and vehemently objected to the proposal for group practice. The minority, however, was willing to accept hospital insurance plans provided they were sponsored and controlled by organized medicine. Its view in general coincided with the emerging view of the AMA. The hostility with which the majority report was greeted by the medical profession is evident from the pages of the *Journal of the American Medical Association* which labeled it as "inciting to revolution." The words of the then-editor of the *Journal*, Dr. Morris Fishbein, indicate better than any other statement we could make the racist and antigovernment attitude so characteristic of organized medicine at the time:

> One must review the expenditure of almost a million dollars by the committee and its final report with mingled amusement and regret. A colored boy spent a dollar taking twenty rides on the merry-go-round. When he got off, his mammy said, "Boy, you spent yo' money but where you been?"

This Fishbein felt was the same as the committee's efforts. He even went so far as to call the recommendation for group practice an attempt to establish medical "soviets."[20]

In spite of such vehement opposition, national health insurance became a major issue during the early years of President Franklin D. Roosevelt's administration. The depression, with its resulting desperation, once again created a climate of opinion favorable to social legislation. Many physicians found themselves with rapidly declining incomes and were unable to collect from their out-of-work patients. This helped change their attitudes, at least temporarily. In 1933, Congress, with AMA approval, appropriated money to help pay doctor's fees. This temporary measure was soon found to be inadequate. To deal more effectively with this and other problems, President Roosevelt in 1934 appointed a cabinet-level Committee on Economic Security under the chairmanship of Frances Perkins, Secretary of Labor. Mrs. Perkins immediately announced that she favored enacting into law substantially all of the social insurance measures which European countries earlier had set up. Harry Hopkins, who held various jobs under Roosevelt and acted as his close adviser, was also in favor of health insurance. The omens seemed favorable but by the time the committee completed its report the AMA had once again announced its opposition to health insurance. Fearful that medical opposition would prevent the passage of any social security legislation, Roosevelt requested the House Ways and Means Committee to strike most provisions dealing with medical care from the bill establishing Social Security. With these deletions, Social Security was enacted into law. Token concession to health insurance supporters was given in the form of increased grants-in-aid to states for maternal and infant preventive care and a strengthened public health program, and both of these measures were passed over the opposition of the AMA.

The extent to which organized medicine was prepared to go was demonstrated by the case of the Milbank Fund, set up by Albert G. Milbank, chairman of the Borden Company. The Milbank Fund had granted money for local studies of preventive medicine, and its secretary, John A. Kingsbury, had criticized the AMA for its opposition to the then-pending Social Security bill. A number of medical journals began hinting through editorials that a boycott of Borden products would have a salutary effect on the fund. Not surprisingly, doctors' recommendations of Borden's irradiated evaporated milk for babies fell off and so did company profits. Milbank was led to deny his fund had ever endorsed compulsory health insurance or "any other plan to distribute the costs of medical care." Shortly afterwards, Kingsbury lost his post as secretary of the fund.

In spite of such actions, the leaders of the AMA realized there was a growing demand for some kind of health insurance. To head off any government-sponsored plan they reversed their opposition to voluntary insurance plans. The first to gain support were the hospital plans, particularly the Blue Cross, which had its origin at Baylor University in Texas in 1929. By 1935 hospitals had enrolled some 23,000 people in more than 400 different employee groups. In 1933 the American Hospital Association's Board of Trustees approved the principle of hospital insurance as a practical solution to the more equitable distribution of the costs of hospital care. The American College of Surgeons, whose members were dependent upon hospitals, endorsed a similar scheme in spite of AMA opposition. By 1937 the American Hospital Association had taken to approving various hospital plans which met its criteria by allowing such plans to use its trademark of the blue cross. In the first list of Blue Cross subscribers published in 1938, some million and a half people were enrolled. By 1953 some 41.8 million persons were enrolled in Blue Cross plans.

Hospital insurance was one thing, prepaid medical care was quite another. Here the opposition of the AMA was much more vigorous. The matter came to a head in the case of the Group Health Association established in 1937 in Washington D.C. by employees of the Federal Home Owners Loan Corporation. This nonprofit prepayment hospitalization and medical care program contracted with physicians to serve its members. The doctors employed by the group soon found themselves expelled from the District of Columbia Medical Society and barred from the seven district hospitals because of their lack of AMA certification. The District Medical Society even went so far as to warn physicians of a rule barring medical consultations with nonsociety members. Hospitals were also warned that if they accepted patients from the group they would lose the AMA approval for their intern-training programs. The effect of such action was to deny hospitalization to members of the Group Health Association. Because of these and other "criminal actions" against the health group, the United States Government instituted a suit for criminal violation against the American Medical Association and the District of Columbia Medical Society. The resulting conviction was eventually affirmed by the United States Supreme Court in 1943. In the meantime, to head off any similar plans, the AMA set up a Council of Medical Service and Public Relations designed to encourage state medical societies to make some type of health insurance plans available to the public, something which several state medical societies had already initiated. To coordinate these plans, Associated Medical Care Plans was created in 1945 and adopted the Blue Shield as its copyrighted symbol.[21]

Medicare

The goal of a national health insurance was still a lingering dream, at least to some. In 1939 a national health proposal was finally introduced into the United States Senate by Robert F. Wagner of New York. It failed to get out of committee, but Wagner continued to introduce it in successive sessions. In 1943 he was joined by Senator James Murray and Representative John Dingell and in this and subsequent years it was known as the Wagner-Murray-Dingell bill. In spite of public opinion polls indicating strong national support for governmentally sponsored health insurance, the AMA and its allies were able to prevent the bill from coming to a vote.[22] After repeated failures to secure a vote, health reformers decided to concentrate on a lesser goal, health benefits for social security beneficiaries. This concept had great appeal because the financial drain of serious illness was the most devastating for the elderly and for the welfare recipient, and it was these groups which were the least likely to be covered by voluntary insurance plans. Moreover, the growing percentage and numbers of the elderly in the population represented a politically potent interest group. In 1957 Congressman Aime J. Forand of Rhode Island introduced a bill to furnish hospital, surgical, and nursing benefits to all social security beneficiaries. Opposition sprang almost immediately from the AMA, the National Chamber of Commerce, the National Association of Manufacturers, the Health Insurance Association, the Pharmaceutical Association, and the American Farm Bureau Federation. Support came from organized labor, from the National Association of Social Workers, the National Farmers Union, and, most importantly, the American Nurses Association. The nurses' support was important because it indicated that a significant number of health professionals were opposed to the AMA stand. The support of the nurses was also a factor in encouraging the American Hospital Association to reevaluate its position on health insurance. Though the AHA did not at this time come out in support, it did not oppose the bill, and the association took the opportunity to point out that something had to be done to help elderly patients pay their bills if only because so many hospitals were being left with uncollectable debts.

In 1960 Senator Robert Kerr of Oklahoma and Congressman Wilbur Mills of Arkansas introduced a substitute bill providing for federal subsidies to states in order to help pay for the health care of welfare recipients, including aged indigents. Though this was a weak compromise for the Forand bill, it had the merit of being enacted. The new legislation soon proved to be ineffective because many states never bothered to institute the programs necessary to utilize the grants. In 1962 the Medicare bill, a revision of the original Forand bill, was again introduced but this time it had the full support of the President, John F. Kennedy. Although it failed to get out of committee in that session of Congress it gathered support and was enacted into law in 1965 under President Lyndon B. Johnson.[2 3]

Financed through the social security system, Medicare provides two separate but coordinated coverages: hospital insurance for most persons aged 65 or over and supplemental medical insurance for those persons in the same age group who voluntarily enroll and pay the required monthly premiums. Although the patients are required to pay a portion of their hospital bill, the coverage is substantial. A companion bill, upgrading the provisions of the Kerr-Mills bill, was also passed in that year and is generally known under the term Medicaid, although various states call it by different terms. It gave funds to states to set up health care programs for welfare recipients covered under the federal programs for families with needy children, the totally or partially blind, and the totally disabled. In order to cut down medical opposition and that of the insurance lobby, Medicare was administered through voluntary insurance carriers, usually Blue Cross. More troublesome was the fact that little control was put over the fees, and one of the immediate results of the passage of Medicare and Medicaid was the escalation of doctors' fees, something which was predicted by almost everyone who had ever studied medical care delivery systems. Hospital costs also skyrocketed, although the connection of these increases to the legislation is due more to past practices than any new ones. The health industry has never been a particularly efficient one and the lack of government controls did little to encourage economy.

The Current Situation

In spite of these improvements in the medical care delivery system, health care remains in a crisis simply because it still is not organized to meet the needs of today. In fact, the very opposition of the organized medical profession to past health schemes has so changed American medicine that programs such as Medicare, which fail to take these changes into account, are bound to be in difficulty. The reluctance of physicians to accept medical insurance led more and more of the medical plans to concentrate upon hospital insurance. Most such hospital plans were made on a cost-plus basis, which meant that hospitals were free to expand or buy new equipment to meet needs, both anticipated and hoped-for. Hospitals were able to do this because the costs, almost any costs in fact, would be automatically covered by insurance. Moreover, the opposition of physicians to health insurance led more and more medical activities to be put into the hospital in order to gain reimbursement for the patient, and in the process, the physician became more and more dependent upon the hospital. Activities which in an earlier period were carried out in the physician's office now were done in the hospital in order for the patient to be reimbursed for his expenditures. Hospitals became a place not only for the sick or injured but for patients undergoing diagnostic work as the doctor knew the only way the patient could have his insurance company pay was to put him into the hospital.

At the same time the nature of medical education in the United States changed, mainly because the federal government poured billions of dollars into biomedical research. In fact, so much money was available that the central activity of the country's major medical schools changed from teaching medical students to carrying out medical research. This not only tremendously increased the cost of medical education both to the individual and to the taxpayer, but in the process it also erected an ever-escalating ladder of medical costs. For example, during the 10-year period from 1959 to 1969 the budget for the Stanford University School of Medicine rose from $5.7 million to $25.5 million without any basic increase in the number of students being graduated. During the same period, federal grants rose from $2.3 million to $15 million or from 41 to 60 percent of the budget; yet the total cost to Stanford, to its students, and to its patients also rose. The bulk of this increase went not to patient care, but to research—until in 1970 Stanford had 375 full-time faculty members and only 357 medical students.[24] It also had several hundred part-time faculty members who came in occasionally for consultation or who maintained a university connection for prestige reasons. The availability of federal funds for medical research had created new glamour positions in medicine for the university medical professors.

In the process, university affiliation has also become a matter of great importance to hospitals who want to attract interns and residents for their ongoing medical care. In New York City, for example, over the past two decades almost all the hospitals and health centers have affiliated with one of the city's seven medical schools. In Baltimore, Johns Hopkins Medical College, and in Boston, Harvard, are the medical centers from which affiliations radiate out to nearby hospitals. The resulting medical empires, networks of affiliated institutions, are replacing the individual hospital as the basic unit of practice just as hospitals earlier replaced the private doctor's office.

Increasingly also major medical institutions have begun to display an internal dynamic of their own, expanding to larger and larger proportions through more and more affiliations in order to maintain their status and their prestige. In the process of building these medical empires, however, the whole nature of patient care has been downgraded because the rewards come from other directions. The result has been what some have called a medical industrial complex. In 1969 Americans spent more than 60 billion dollars on medical care, which represented an 11 percent increase over the previous year and double the amount spent in 1960. The 1969 expenditure amounted to 6.7 percent of the gross national product, which is almost double the percentage spent in other industrialized countries. The health industry is big business, and despite the fact that much of its claims to be nonprofit, it reported some $2.5 billion in after-tax profits. The implications for health care become obvious. Community hospitals, for instance, spent 16 percent more money in 1968 than in 1967 but provided only 3.3 percent more days of inpatient care and 3.7 percent more outpatient visits. While some of the increase went for wages, most of it went to pay the inflated costs of drugs, supplies, and equipment, and in many cases to profits for doctors and to the hospitals. Much of the equipment which was purchased had a planned obsolescence, and in many of the smaller hospitals, such equipment, particularly of the electronic variety, largely went unused. A high proportion of the new building went for research facilities rather than to those devoted to patient care. Inevitably the cost of medical care has increased. In 1950 the nation spent 3.8 billion on hospital care, by 1965 the figure had risen to 13.8 billion, and in 1969—three years after Medicare and Medicaid—expenditures for hospital care alone were running at $20 billion a year.[25] Without materially serving a larger number of patients, county hospitals have also found their costs mounting. The city of Chicago, for example, has seen public expenditures for health care go up fourfold between 1960 and 1970, from $100 million to $400 million, but there is still a major crisis of unmet needs. In 1970 it cost $104 a day just to keep a patient in Cook County Hospital.[26]

Extension of Government-Supported Medical Care

The escalating crisis in medical care has led an increasing number of people publicly to advocate some form of national health insurance. So great is the need, in fact, that most experts are predicting the enactment of some sort of comprehensive medical program within the decade.[27] Although a single well-thought-out health care package might be the ideal way of solving the growing problems, political realities would indicate that reform is more likely to come about in a piecemeal fashion. From this perspective the 1965 Medicare and Medicaid legislation can be viewed as opening wedges in the gradual reform process. The difficulty with the piecemeal system, however, is that long-range goals are too often neglected and for any system to be effective, no matter how it is enacted, it is essential that long-range goals be established.

In our minds one of the most important long-range objectives should be the establishment of a comprehensive health care system, something which is now almost totally lacking in American medicine. This was not true so much in the past, but in recent decades the patchwork financing system and the growing trend toward specialization in medicine have created a fragmentation of care. Though poor people and minorities can now receive a certain amount of health care, the value of the care is not so great as it could be because of fragmentation. The federal government, for example, furnishes care through various agencies to many people—including the aged, the blind, the totally disabled, families with dependent children, veterans, and members of the armed forces. As we have indicated, research hospitals sometimes give outstanding care to a patient with a rare disease or someone who fits into a given study sample, but other seriously ill patients are ignored. Private funds sometimes finance the care of a specific disease, but often these specialized agencies or hospitals are located far from the point of need. Health departments give preventive care to mothers and infants but usually do not give acute care. This maze of eligibility categories is difficult enough for the expert to comprehend, but it is truly formidable for the poor, the uneducated, and those with a language barrier. Moreover, even when services are available in scattered specialty facilities, someone with multiple health problems often must travel around to various specialists because there is no one worker who looks at the total health problem of the patient or evaluates the total regimen. This is true in private-patient care as well as in charitable or governmental medical care.

Any effective plan to deal with health care has to do away with the complex eligibility rules and simply give health care to all of the people, employed or unemployed, rich or poor, citizen or alien, young or old. Health care, in effect, has to be conceptualized as a right for all instead of a privilege for those who have money or accidentally qualify under some special program. We also need to establish some means by which one worker can take the primary responsibility for coordinating the patient's care. In the past this was the role of the general practitioner, but because of the trend in medical education away from producing family doctors and toward gathering ever-more-specialized knowledge, it is possible that the primary care role will fall to a less expensive worker such as the nurse practitioner or the physician's assistant. This worker, whether he be a general practitioner, nurse practitioner, or physician's assistant, should be allowed to treat the less complex illnesses and refer the problems to the various specialists. He should also coordinate the care so that the welfare of the total patient is not overlooked as the specialists narrow focus on diseases or organs.

A second important goal in the establishment of a plan for health care is for the system to be economically feasible. This means that the already existing Medicare-Medicaid legislation needs revision to cut out its inflationary characteristics that have increased costs but not necessarily improved medical care. Fee controls and cost-accounting procedures are badly needed and the unnecessary administrative cost of using intermediate carriers, such as Blue Cross, to do the work the government can do cheaper itself, should be eliminated. Planning for economy is always a difficult aspect of reform because each of the various lobbies works to see that its group gains economic advantages, but it is a crucial step in order to make a health plan workable in the long run.

Both of these major objectives, that of making health care comprehensive and making it economically efficient can, in our minds, best be furthered by the encouragement of government-sponsored health maintenance organizations. Basically these organizations are a form of group practice, something pioneered by Americans. The first group practice was the famed Mayo Clinic in Rochester, Minnesota, in which the various professional and paraprofessional groups work together to treat the patient. The Mayo Clinic, which dates from the 19th century, was originally developed not for preventive reasons but to deal with the seriously ill patient. Its example has been followed by various other specialized clinics such as the Cleveland Clinic, the Ochsner Clinic in New Orleans, and the Lahey Clinic in Boston. The consultation of the experts assembled in these clinics probably furnishes the best medical care in the world. These "clinics" had little opposition from organized medicine but when the concept of the clinic was combined with the prepaid factor and opened up to a wider public, organized medicine went into opposition. In fact, many states, on the urging of their medical associations, passed laws prohibiting group practice of any kind and such laws still exist in several states.

The two best-known of the prepaid group practice insurance plans are the Health Insurance Plan (HIP) in New York and Kaiser-Permanente on the West Coast. Both have the advantage of adjusting to the realities of the way in which the best medicine is increasingly practiced in this country and they have the additional advantage of costing less than other insurance plans. Kaiser-Permanente was started by Henry J. Kaiser, the California contractor, as a plan for his employees when he was building Grand Coulee Dam. It was expanded during World War II as he turned to building ships, and then further expanded as the industrialist turned to manufacturing steel, aluminum, and automobiles. Shortly after the end of the war the system went public and through contracts with various unions and other organizations Kaiser-Permanente began offering total prepaid medical care to all subscribers.[28] For those who belong to the more complete Kaiser plans everything is paid except for drugs used in outpatient care, and these are sold at less than wholesale prices. From the first, Kaiser-Permanente has insisted that all companies and organizations offering their plan also offer competing ones. This has tended to keep subscribers from feeling trapped within the Kaiser system, and it has also served as an effective cost-accounting procedure. The great virtue of the Kaiser system, and that of similar ones, is that they emphasize preventive medicine. The difference that effective preventive care makes was demonstrated by a study of federal employees on the West Coast, some of whom were insured by Kaiser-Permanente and others by Blue Cross-Blue Shield. The study found that although Kaiser subscribers had greater contact with physicians and other health practitioners they spent far less time in the hospital. Each unit of 1,000 federal employees spent a total of 433 days in a hospital per year under the Kaiser plan while those under Blue Cross-Blue Shield spent an average of 865 days per 1,000 employees. This enabled Kaiser to keep its costs some 20 percent lower than in California's voluntary hospitals and to keep the rate of increase to less than half of the national rate.

Prepaid group plans achieve these lower costs by practicing effective preventive medicine and cutting out unnecessary operations or other medical procedures. Kaiser surgery rates, for example, were little more than one half of the Blue Cross figures. As one Kaiser official stated, Kaiser has a vested interest in keeping the patient well—a few pennies spent on prevention saves dollars spent on the cure. Kaiser physicians and employees are salaried, but those at the higher levels are also eligible to become partners and as such are eligible to share in the profits from the plan. In a 1966 study of various prepaid group practice plans, it was found that doctors in group practice performed fewer than one-quarter the number of tonsillectomies for each 1,000 enrollees, half the number of appendectomies, and only slightly more than half of the hysterectomies done by fee-for-service physicians. This same trend appeared with those welfare patients enrolled in group practice plans. In 1962, for example, New York City's HIP undertook to treat welfare recipients and it was found that its physicians made but one-quarter the number of premium-priced home calls and ordered but one-half the highly profitable (and highly expensive) laboratory tests which fee-for-service, solo practitioners were accustomed to require.[29]

Under a national health insurance plan, such health maintenance organizations would contract to care for a given number of patients for an annual fee rather than being paid for each service that is rendered.[30] The American health maintenance group would undoubtedly be a more effective capitation plan than the panels used in England primarily because the primary practitioners in the American plan would not be separated from the collaboration and stimulation of the specialists as they are in England.

This book is not the place to decide how any national health plan is financed. Such a topic deserves a study in its own right. It still is possible, however, to speculate, if only briefly. An insurance principle in which each worker contributes a portion of his salary as is done under Social Security seems a likely possibility. Although payment out of general revenues, which receive a greater share from higher income levels in society, would be easier for the marginal worker to afford it would be more difficult to get through Congress. Probably some combination of these two sources of financing is the most pragmatic suggestion we have to offer.

Any long-range planning for health reform also requires that consideration be given to better utilization of health workers. One of the most obvious consequences of any extension of medical care will be the need for more health workers. One of the easiest ways to solve the problem is to make more effective use of present workers. Laws which bar workers from performing tasks which they can safely and effectively perform need to be reconsidered and perhaps repealed. A simple increase in the number of doctors if present trends in medicine continue will not be enough because the present organization of medical schools, with their emphasis on research and specialization, simply accentuates the shortage of physicians. It might well be that financial incentives now being used to encourage research should be reconsidered. Some of the funds might better be spent to educate more doctors of the general-practitioner types, as well as nurses and other health workers who can give actual patient care. The suggestion of the Carnegie Foundation that medical education be shortened also has merit.[31] Care must be taken to see that as the health care industry expands there will not be large numbers of people trapped at the bottom of the economic ladder in the no-advancement jobs such as those of nurses' aides or orderlies. Many such workers are at near-poverty levels of income, which in itself is not a healthy phenomenon. More important, however, is the fact that workers who are trapped with no chance for advancement tend over the years to lose interest in their jobs. Unless some means can be found to interest them in helping to deliver better health care, all the best laid plans of scholarly investigators and government planners will fail. It is not only that these workers should be paid more but they should be given in-service training and encouraged to work to the full level of their capacity. There needs to be a democratization of the health care team. Another obvious answer seems to be the establishment of a career ladder, that is, on-the-job training for advancement with entry points at various levels of the career ladder. This would require greater cooperation between colleges or universities and the health care institutions than now exists, but it would follow current trends. Individuals who first begin as health aides might well gain sufficient experience and education to become practical nurses and even registered nurses. Nurses, on the other hand, should extend their role to cover some of the tasks now done by the fast-disappearing general practitioners. Pharmacists could be better used to back up the physicians in prescribing drugs, either giving advice on their own or working with the group of physicians to indicate what a drug will or will not do instead of having the physician depend upon the drug salesman or detail man for his information. In effect, the pharmacist, the nurse, and the aide should be better utilized and encouraged to develop and use new skills.[32]

Concluding Comments

In this book we have tried to present the health care problems of the major ethnic minority groups in perspective. Although poverty is probably the most crucial variable in the genesis of these problems, there are still many subtle and not so subtle forms of discrimination operating in the health field. Unfortunately, discrimination in other aspects of American life also has consequences for health and in turn poor health helps to perpetuate the cycle of alienation and poverty. We have tried to emphasize that there are no simple solutions, but that the problems come together into a kind of Gordian knot. There are, however, rational and possible steps to take to cut that knot, including (1) eliminating poverty, (2) effectively enforcing the laws against discrimination, and (3) revising our health care delivery system to provide total coverage for all of the people. To some these might seem utopian steps, but until we take effective action against these barriers America will not fully live up to its potential in the health field.

Notes

1. In *Costs and Delivery of Health Services to Older Americans*, Hearings Before the Subcommittee on Health of the Elderly of the Special Committee on Aging, United States Senate, Ninetieth Congress, 1st Session, Part I (Washington, D.C.: U.S. Government Printing Office, 1967), pp. 84-85.
2. Alonzo S. Yerby, "Health Departments, Hospitals and Health Services," mimeographed copy of an address given at the Fiftieth Anniversary Celebration, October 6, 1966, at The Johns Hopkins School of Hygiene and Public Health.

3. Robert L. Heilbroner, "Benign Neglect in the United States," *Trans-Action*, 7, No. 12 (October 1970), pp. 15-22.

4. See, for example, Alvin L. Schorr, "The Case for Federal Welfare," *The Nation* (May 3, 1971), pp. 555-557. Mr. Schorr was a former Deputy Secretary of the Department of Health, Education, and Welfare.

5. U.S. Bureau of Census, *Current Population Reports*, Series P-60, No. 76, "24 Million Americans—Poverty in the United States, 1969," (Washington, D.C.: U.S. Government Printing Office, 1970). See also a preliminary report of the 1970 figures in the *Los Angeles Times*, May 8, 1971, part 6.

6. See Daniel Patrick Moynihan, *Maximum Feasible Misunderstanding: Community Action in the War on Poverty* (New York: The Free Press, 1969).

7. See Frank Riessman, *Strategies Against Poverty* (New York: Random House, 1969), pp. 21-40.

8. Cynthia H. Kelly, "Fighting Poverty in Urban Areas," and "Fighting Poverty in Rural Areas," in *New Directions for Nurses*, edited by Bonnie and Vern Bullough (New York: Springer, 1971), pp. 248-259, 259-266.

9. U.S. Social Security Administration, *Social Security Programs Throughout the World* (Washington, D.C.: U.S. Government Printing Office, 1967).

10. For a popular account of opposition of the AMA see Ed Cray, *In Failing Health: The Medical Crises and the AMA* (Indianapolis: The Bobbs-Merrill Company, 1970),pp. 40-59.

11. William A. Glasser, *Paying the Doctor: System of Remuneration and Their Effects* (Baltimore: The Johns Hopkins Press, 1970), p. 178.

12. Milton I. Roemer, *The Organization of Medical Care Under Social Security* (Geneva: International Labour Office, 1969), pp. 31, 46-47.

13. Glasser, *op. cit.*, pp. 202-203.

14. *Ibid.*, pp. 286-287.

15. Roemer, *The Organization of Medical Care*, pp. 52-55.

16. Glaser, *op. cit.*, pp. 52-53.

17. *Ibid.*, pp. 206-207; Milton I. Roemer, "Highlights of Soviet Health Services," *Milbank Memorial Fund Quarterly*, 15 (No. 4, October 1962), pp. 381-385.

18. Peter A. Corning, *The Evolution of Medicare: From Idea to Law*, Research Report, No. 29 (Washington, D.C.: U.S. Government Printing Office, 1969), pp. 5-16.

19. Committee on the Costs of Medical Care, *Medical Care for the American People* (Chicago: University of Chicago Press, 1932; reprinted by U.S. Government Printing Office, 1970).

20. Cray, *op. cit.*, p. 65.

21. George Rosen, *A History of Public Health* (New York: M D Publications, 1958), pp. 456-462; Vern and Bonnie Bullough, *The Emergence of Modern Nursing* (New York: Macmillan, 1969), pp. 196-198.

22. Social Security Administration, *The Evolution of Medicare*, pp. 53-57.

23. *Ibid.*, pp. 74-115; Cray, *op. cit.*, pp. 90-109.

24. John Walsh, "Stanford School of Medicine (1) Problems over More than Money," *Science* (February 12, 1971), pp. 551-553; see also Vern L. Bullough, "Financial Crisis on the Campus," *Progressive* (October 1971), pp. 37-40.
25. *The American Health Empire: Power, Profits and Politics*, A Health PAC Book prepared by Barbara and John Ehrenreich (New York: Random House, 1970), pp. 96-103.
26. Jack Star, "Cook County Hospital: The Terrible Place," *Look* (May 18, 1971), pp. 24-33.
27. See, for example, Wilbur J. Cohen, "National Health Insurance—Problems and Prospects," the Michael M. Davis Lecture for 1970 at the Center for Health Administration Studies, Graduate School of Business, University of Chicago. Printed in pamphlet form by the University of Chicago, 1970.
28. For a discussion of this and other plans see Herman M. and Anne R. Somers, *Doctors, Patients and Health Insurance: The Organization and Financing of Medical Care* (Washington D.C.: The Brookings Institution, 1961).
29. Cray, *op. cit.*, pp. 190-191; see also Roul Tunley, *The American Health Scandal* (New York: Harper & Row, 1966), pp. 112-125.
30. Paul M. Ellwood, Jr., "Health Maintenance Organizations: Concept and Strategy," *Hospitals*, 45 (March 16, 1971), pp. 53-56.
31. Carnegie Commission on Higher Education, *Higher Education and the Nation's Health: Policies for Dental and Medical Education* (New York: McGraw-Hill, 1970).
32. Bonnie and Vern Bullough, "A Career Ladder in Nursing," *American Journal of Nursing*, 71: 1938-1943, 1971.

Bibliography

Adair, J., and Deuschle, K. W. *The People's Health: Medicine and Anthropology in a Navaho Community* (New York: Appleton-Century-Crofts, 1970).

Addams, J. *Twenty Years at Hull House* (New York: The Macmillan Co., 1912).

Alpert, J., Kosa, J., and Haggerty, R. J. "A Month of Illness and Health Care Among Low Income Families," *Public Health Reports*, 82 (August 1967), pp. 705-713.

American Nurses' Association. *Facts About Nursing* (New York: ANA, 1969).

American Public Health Association. *Evaluatory Study on Operation of the Migrant Health Program Under the Migrant Health Act*, December 30, 1964 (New York: mimeographed), pp. 1-49.

Anderson, E. H., and Lesser, A. J. "Maternity Care in the United States: Gains and Gaps," *American Journal of Nursing*, 66 (July 1966), pp. 1539-1544.

Baca, J. "Some Health Beliefs of the Spanish Speaking," *American Journal of Nursing*, 69 (October 1969), pp. 2172-2176.

Badgley, R. F., and Wolfe, S. *Doctors' Strike: Medical Care and Conflict in Saskatchewan* (New York: Atherton Press, Inc., 1967).

Barron, M. L. *Minorities in a Changing World* (New York: Alfred A. Knopf, 1967).

Bennett, F. "The Condition of Farm Workers," in *Poverty in America*, edited by Louis A. Ferman, Joyce L. Karnbluh, and Alan Haber (Ann Arbor: University of Michigan Press, revised edition, 1968), pp. 303-314.

Bergner, L., and Yerby, A. S. "Low Income and Barriers to Use of Health Service," *New England Journal of Medicine*, 278 (March 7, 1968), pp. 541-546.

Berle, B. B. *Eighty Puerto Rican Families in New York City: Health and Disease Studied in Context* (New York: Columbia University Press, 1958).

Bigham, G. D. "To Communicate with Negro Patients," *American Journal of Nursing*, 64 (September 1964), pp. 113-115.

Birch, H. G., and Gussow, J. D. *Disadvantaged Children: Health, Nutrition and School Failure* (New York: Harcourt, Brace & World, 1970).

Blau, P. M., and Duncan, O. D. *The American Occupational Structure* (New York: John Wiley, 1967).

Blum, R., et al. *Society and Drugs; Social and Cultural Observations*, Vol. 1 (San Francisco: Jossey-Bass, 1969).

Bogardus, E. S. The Mexican in the United States (New York: Arno Press, 1934; republished, 1970).

Bongarts, R. "Who Am I? The Indian Sickness," *The Nation* (April 27, 1970), pp. 496-498.

Breed, W. "Suicide, Migration and Race: A Study of Cases in New Orleans," *The Journal of Social Issues*, 22 (January 1966), pp. 30-43.

Brown, C. *Manchild in the Promised Land* (New York: The Macmillan Company, 1965).

Brown, H. J. "Changes in the Delivery of Health Care," *American Journal of Nursing*, 68 (November 1968), pp. 2362-2364.

Brown, L. "Hunger USA: The Public Pushes Congress," *Journal of Health and Social Behavior*, 11 (June 1970), pp. 115-126.

Bullock, P. *Watts: The Aftermath* (New York: Grove Press, 1969).

Bullough, B. "Alienation and School Segregation," *Integrated Education*, in press, 1972.

Bullough, B. "Alienation in the Ghetto," *American Journal of Sociology*, 72 (March 1967), pp. 469-478.

Bullough, B. "Malnutrition Among Egyptian Infants," *Nursing Research*, 18 (Spring 1969), p. 172.

Bullough, B. *Social-Psychological Barriers to Housing Desegregation* (Los Angeles: University of California, Graduate School of Business Administration, 1969).

Bullough, B., and Bullough, V. "A Career Ladder in Nursing," *American Journal of Nursing*, 71: 1938-1943, 1971.

Bullough, B. and Bullough, V. *New Directions for Nurses* (New York: Springer, 1971).

Bullough, B. and Bullough, V. *Issues in Nursing* (New York: Springer, 1966).

Bullough, V., and Bullough, B. *Emergence of Modern Nursing* 2nd edition (New York: The Macmillan Company, 1969).

Bullough, V., and Bullough, B. *The Untouchables* (Chicago: Committee Against Discrimination and the Southern Conference on Education, 1955).

Bullough, V., and Bullough, B. *What Color Are Your Germs?* (Chicago: The Committee To End Discrimination in Chicago Medical Institutions, 1955).

Bullough, V. "Financial Crisis on the Campus," *Progressive* (October, 1971), pp. 37-41.

Bureau of Maternal and Child Health, California State Department of Public Health. *Health for the Harvesters: A Ten Year Report by the Farm Workers Health Service* (State of California, 1970).

Burgess, E. W. "Urban Areas," *Chicago: An Experiment in Social Science Research*, edited by T. V. Smith and L. White (Chicago: University of Chicago Press, 1929), pp. 113-138.

Cahalan, D., Cisin, I., and Crossley, H. M. *American Drinking Practices: A National Survey of Behavior and Attitudes Related to Alcoholic Beverages*, Social Research Group, George Washington University, Washington, D.C., Report No. 3, 1967.

Cahill, I. D. "The Mother from the Slum Neighborhood," *Current Concepts in Nursing Care* (Columbus, Ohio: Ross Laboratories, 1964).

California Legislative Assembly Committee on Health and Welfare. *Malnutrition: One Key to the Poverty Cycle* (January 1970).

Campbell, A. A. "Fertility and Family Planning Among Non-White Married Couples in the United States," *Eugenics Quarterly*, 12 (September 1961), pp. 124-131.

Carnegie Commission on Higher Education. *Higher Education and the Nation's Health: Policies for Dental and Medical Education* (New York: McGraw-Hill, 1970).

Carnegie, M. E. "Are Negro Schools of Nursing Needed Today?" *Nursing Outlook* 12 (February 1964), pp. 52-56. Reprinted in *New Directions for Nurses*, edited by Bonnie and Vern Bullough (New York: Springer, 1971), pp. 292-303.

Carr-Saunders, A. M. *World Population* (Oxford: Clarendon Press, 1936).

Caudill, H. M. *Night Comes to the Cumberlands: A Biography of a Depressed Area* (Boston: Little, Brown and Co., 1963).

Chapman, C. B., and Talmadge, J. M. "The Evolution of the Right to Health Concept in the United States," *The Pharos of Alpha Omega Alpha*, 34 (January 1971), pp. 30-51.

Chase, H. C. "Perinatal and Infant Mortality in the United States and Six West European Countries," *American Journal of Public Health*, 57 (October 1967), pp. 1735-1748.

Chein, I. "Psychological, Social and Epidemiological Factors in Drug Addiction," *Rehabilitating the Narcotic Addict*, a report of the Institute on New Developments in the Rehabilitation of the Narcotic Addict (Washington, D.C.: U.S. Government Printing Office, 1966), pp. 53-66.

Chenault, L. R. *The Puerto Rican Migrant in New York City* (New York: Columbia University Press, 1938).

"Chinatown, U.S.A., 1970," *California's Health*, 27-8 (February 1970), pp. 1-3.

Civil Rights '63, Report of the United States Commission on Civil Rights (Washington, D.C.: U.S. Government Printing Office, 1963).

Clark, K. B. *Dark Ghetto: Dilemmas of Social Power* (New York: Harper & Row, 1965).

Clark, K. B. *Prejudice and Your Child* (Boston: The Beacon Press, 1955).

Clark, K., and Clark, M. "Emotional Factors in Racial Identification and Preference in Negro Children," in *Mental Health and Segregation*, edited by M. Grossack (New York: Springer, 1963), pp. 53-63.

Clark, M. *Health in the Mexican-American Culture: A Community Study* (Berkeley: University of California Press, 1970).

Cogan, L. *Negroes for Medicine: Report of a Macy Conference* (Baltimore: The Johns Hopkins Press, 1968).

Cohen, W. J. "National Health Insurance—Problems and Prospects," The 1970 Michael M. Davis Lecture for 1970 at the Center for Health Administration Studies, Graduate School of Business, University of Chicago.

Coleman, J. S., Campbell, E. Q., Hobson, C., McPartland, J., Mood, A. M., Weinfield, F. D., and York, R. L. *Equality of Educational Opportunity* (Washington, D.C.: U.S. Office of Education, 1966).

Coleman, J. S. *Resources for Social Change: Race in the United States* (New York: Wiley Interscience, 1971).

Committee on the Costs of Medical Care. *Medical Care for the American People* (Chicago: University of Chicago Press, 1932; reprinted by U.S. Government Printing Office, 1970).

Committee on Labor and Public Welfare, United States Senate, Special Subcommittee on Indian Education. *Indian Education: A National Tragedy—A National Challenge* (Washington, D.C.: U.S. Government Printing Office, 1969).

Cornely, P. B. "The Health Status of the Negro Today and in the Future," *American Journal of Public Health*, 58 (April 1968), pp. 647-654.

Corning, P. A. *The Evolution of Medicare . . . from Idea to Law*, U.S. Department of Health, Education, and Welfare, Social Security Administration, Research Report No. 29 (Washington, D.C.: U.S. Government Printing Office, 1969).

Cray, E. *In Failing Health: The Medical Crisis and the A.M.A.* (Indianapolis: The Bobbs-Merrill Company, 1970).

Crowley, A. E., and Nicholson, H. C. "Negro Enrollment in Medical Schools," *Journal of the American Medical Association*, 210 (October 6, 1969), pp. 96-100.

Cuban Refugee Problem, a report of the Hearings Before the Subcommittee to Investigate Problems Connected with Refugees and Escapees, Committee on the Judiciary, United States Senate, in three parts (Washington, D.C.: U.S. Government Printing Office, 1966).

Cuba's Children in Exile: The Story of the Unaccompanied Cuban Refugee Children's Program (published by the Children's Bureau of the U.S. Department of Health, Education, and Welfare, 1967).

Deasy, L. C. "Socio-Economic Status and Participation in the Poliomyelitis Vaccine Trial," *American Sociological Review*, 21 (April 1956), pp. 185-191.

Delgado, G., Brumback, C. L., and Deaver, M. B. "Eating Patterns Among Migrant Families," *Public Health Reports*, 76 (April 1961), pp. 349-355.

Deutsch, M., Katz, I., and Jensen, A. R., editors. *Social Class, Race and Psychological Development* (New York: Holt, Rinehart & Winston, 1968).

Division of Indian Health, Program Analysis and Special Studies Branch, *Eskimos, Indians and Aleuts of Alaska*, part of U.S. Department of Health, Education, and Welfare Report, *Indians on Federal Reservations* (Washington, D.C.: U.S. Government Printing Office, 1963).

Dohrenwend, B. P., and Dohrenwend, B. S. *Social Status and Psychological Disorder: A Causal Inquiry* (New York: Wiley-Interscience, 1969).

Dorson, N. *Discrimination and Civil Rights* (Boston: Little, Brown and Company, 1969).

Douglas, J. *The Social Meaning of Suicide* (Princeton: Princeton University Press Co., 1967).

Dublin, L. I. *Suicide: A Sociological and Statistical Study* (New York: Ronald Press, 1963).

Duff, R. S., and Hollingshead, A. B. *Sickness and Society* (New York: Harper & Row, 1968).

Dumas, R. G. "This I Believe ... About Nursing and the Poor," *Nursing Outlook*, 17 (September 1969), pp. 47-49.

Dummett, C. O. *The Growth and Development of the Negro in Dentistry* (Chicago: The Stanek Press for the National Dental Association, 1952).

Dunham, H. W. *Community and Schizophrenia: An Epidemiological Analysis* (Detroit: Wayne State University Press, 1965).

Durkheim, E. *Suicide: A Study in Sociology*, translated from the French by John A. Spaulding and George Simpson (Glencoe, Ill.: Free Press, 1951).

Dworkis, M. B., editor. *The Impact of Puerto Rican Migration on Governmental Services in New York City* (New York: New York University Press, 1957).

"Educational Preparation for Nursing–1969," *Nursing Outlook*, 18 (September 1970), pp. 52-57.

Ehrenreich, B., and Ehrenreich, J. *The American Health Empire: Power, Profits and Politics*, A Health PAC Book (New York: Random House, 1970).

Eilers, R. D. "National Health Insurance: What Kind and How Much," *New England Journal of Medicine*, 284:945-954, 1971.

Ellwood, P. M. "Health Maintenance Organizations: Concept and Strategy," *Hospitals*, 45 (March 16, 1971), pp. 53-56.

Elman, R. M. *The Poorhouse State: The American Way of Life on Public Assistance* (New York: A Delta Book, 1966).

Fagen, R. R., Brody, R. A., and O'Leary, T. J. *Cubans in Exile: Disaffection and the Revolution* (Stanford: Stanford University Press, 1968).

Falk, I. S. "Beyond Medicare," *American Journal of Public Health*, 59 (April 1969), pp. 608-619.

Falkner, F. *Key Issues in Infant Mortality, Report of a Conference April 16-18, 1969, Washington, D.C.* (Washington, D.C.: U.S. Government Printing Office, 1969).

Faris, R. E. L., and Dunham, H. W. *Mental Disorders in Urban Areas: An*

Ecological Study of Schizophrenia and Other Psychoses (Chicago: University of Chicago Press, 1939).

Ferenczi, I. *International Migrations, Volume 1, Statistics* (New York: Arno Press, 1929; republished, 1970).

Fey, H. E., and McNickel, D. *Indians and Other Americans: Two Ways of Life* (New York: Harper & Brothers, 1959).

Filer, J. L. "The United States Today—Is it Free of Public Health Nutrition Problems Today?—Anemia," presented to the American Public Health Association, Miami Beach, Florida, October 24, 1967; cited in *Hunger, U.S.A.*

Fogelson, R. M., and Hill, R. B. "Who Riots? A Study of Participation in the 1967 Riots," in *Supplemental Studies for the National Advisory Commission on Civil Disorders*, Chairman, Otto Kerner (Washington, D.C.: U.S. Government Printing Office, 1968).

Forbes, J. D., editor. *The Indian in America's Past* (Englewood Cliffs, N.J.: Prentice-Hall, 1964).

Ford, T. R., editor. *The Southern Appalachian Region: A Survey* Lexington: University of Kentucky Press, 1962).

Foster, G. M. "Relationships Between Spanish and Spanish-American Folk Medicine," *Journal of American Folklore*, 66 (1953), pp. 201-217.

Frackelton, D. L., and Faville, K. "Opportunities in Nursing for Disadvantaged Youth," *Nursing Outlook* (April 1966), pp. 26-28.

Franklin, J. H. *From Slavery to Freedom* (New York: Alfred A. Knopf, 1967).

Frazier, E. F. *Black Bourgeoisie* (New York: Collier Books, 1962).

Frazier, E. F. *The Negro Family in the United States* (Chicago: University of Chicago, 1939).

Freedman, R., Whelpton, P. K., and Campbell, A. A. *Family Planning, Sterility and Population Growth* (New York: McGraw-Hill, 1959).

Freidson, E. "Client Control and Medical Practice," *American Journal of Sociology*, 65 (1960), pp. 374-382.

Freidson, E. *Patient's View of Medical Practice* (New York: Russell Sage Foundation, 1961).

Friedson, E. *Professional Dominance: The Social Structure of Medical Care* (New York: Atherton Press, 1970).

Furman, S. S., Sweat, L. G., and Crocetti, G. M. "Social Class Factors in the Flow of Children to Outpatient Psychiatric Facilities," *American Journal of Public Health*, 55 (March 1965), pp. 385-392.

Galarza, E., Gallegos, H., and Samora, J. *Mexican-Americans in the Southwest* (Santa Barbara: McNally and Loftin, in cooperation with the Anti-Defamation League of B'nai B'rith, 1969).

Geiger, H. J. "The Endlessly Revolving Door," *American Journal of Nursing* (November 1969), pp. 2435-2445.

Gibbs, J. P. *Suicide* (New York: Harper & Row, 1968).

Gibbs, J. P., and Martin, W. T. *Status Integration and Suicide* (Eugene, Ore.: University of Oregon, 1964).

Gibson, C. D. "The Neighborhood Health Center: The Primary Unit of Health Care," *American Journal of Public Health*, 58 (July 1968), pp. 1188-1191.

Ginzberg, E., with Ostow, M. *Men, Money and Medicine* (New York: Columbia University Press, 1969).

Glaser, W. A. *Paying the Doctor: Systems of Remuneration and Their Effects* (Baltimore: The Johns Hopkins Press, 1970).

Glazer, N., and Moynihan, D. P. *Beyond the Melting Pot: The Negroes, Puerto Ricans, Jews, Italians and Irish of New York City* (Cambridge, Mass.: The M.I.T. Press, second edition, 1970).

Goffman, E. *Asylums: Essays on the Social Situation of Mental Patients and Other Inmates* (New York: Anchor Books, 1961).

Goldscheider, C., and Uhlenberg, P. R. "Minority Group Status and Fertility," *American Journal of Sociology*, 74 (January 1969), pp. 361-372.

Goldschmid, M. L., editor. *Black Americans and White Racism, Theory and Research* (New York: Holt, Rinehart & Winston, 1970).

Goldstein, M. S. "Longevity and Health Status of the Negro American," *Journal of Negro Education*, 32 (Fall 1963), pp. 337-348.

Goode, E. *The Marijuana Smokers* (New York: Basic Books, 1970).

Goode, E., editor. *Marijuana* (New York: Atherton Press, 1969).

Goode, W. J. "Illegitimacy in the Caribbean Social Structure," *American Sociological Review*, 25 (February 1960), pp. 21-30.

Goodman, M. E. *Race Awareness in Young Children* (Cambridge, Mass.: Addison-Wesley Press, 1952).

Gordon, M. *Assimilation in American Life: The Role of Race, Religion, and National Origin* (New York: Oxford University Press, 1964).

Gossett, T. F. *Race: The History of an Idea in America* (Dallas: Southern Methodist University Press, 1963).

Gottesman, I. I. "Biogenetics of Race and Class," in *Social Class, Race and Psychological Development*, edited by M. Deutsch, I. Katz, and A. R. Jensen (New York: Holt, Rinehart & Winston, 1968), pp. 11-51.

Gray, R. M., Kesler, J. P., and Moody, P. M. "The Effects of Social Class and Friends' Expectations on Oral Polio Vaccination Participation," *American Journal of Public Health*, 56 (December 1966), pp. 2028-2032.

Grebler, L., Moore, J. W., and Guzman, R. C. *The Mexican-American People: The Nation's Second Largest Minority* (New York: The Free Press, 1970).

Greenberg, S. *The Quality of Mercy: A Report on the Critical Condition of Hospital and Medical Care in America* (New York: Atheneum, 1971).

Greer, C. "Public Schools: The Myth of the Melting Pot," *Saturday Review* (November 15, 1969), pp. 84-86, 102-103.

Grey, A. L. ed. *Class and Personality in Society* (New York: Atherton Press, 1969).

Grier, W. H., and Cobbs, P. M. *Black Rage* (New York: Basic Books, 1968).

Groat, H. T., and Neal, A. G. "Social Psychological Correlates of Urban Fertility," *American Sociological Review*, 32 (December 1967), pp. 945-959.

Grossack, M. M. *Mental Health and Segregation* (New York: Springer, 1963).

Gunter, L. M. "The Effects of Segregation on Nursing Students," *Nursing Outlook*, 9 (February 1961), pp. 74-76.

Gutelius, M. F. "The Problem of Iron Deficiency Anemia in Preschool Negro Children," *American Journal of Public Health*, 59 (February 1969), pp. 290-295.

Haefner, D. P., Kegeles, S. S., Kirscht, J., and Rosenstock, I. M. "Preventive Actions in Dental Disease, Tuberculosis and Cancer," *Public Health Reports*, 82 (May 1967), pp. 451-459.

Hagan, W. T. *American Indians* (Chicago: University of Chicago, 1961).

Hammond, E. I. "Studies in Fetal and Infant Mortality. II—Differentials in Mortality by Sex and Race," *American Journal of Public Health*, 55 (August 1965), pp. 1152-1163.

Handler, O. *The Uprooted* (Boston: Atlantic Little, Brown, 1952).

Harrington, M. *The Other America: Poverty in the United States* (Baltimore: Penguin Books, 1962).

Harris, L. "How the Poor View Their Health," in *Sources: A Blue Cross Report of Health Problems of the Poor* (Chicago: Blue Cross Association, 1968), pp. 21-36.

Harris, Senator and Mrs. F. R. "Indian Health," in *Sources: A Blue Cross Report of Health Problems of the Poor* (Chicago: Blue Cross Association, 1968), pp. 38-43.

Harris, S. E. *The Economics of American Medicine* (New York: The Macmillan Company, 1964).

Harvey, L. H. "Educational Problems of Minority Group Nurses," *Nursing Outlook*, 18 (September 1970), pp. 43-50.

Haynes, A. M. "Distribution of Black Physicians in the United States," *Journal of the American Medical Association*, 210 (October 6, 1969), pp. 93-95.

Health Advisory Committee to the Appalachian Regional Commission. *Report*, March 1966.

"Health Care: What the Poor People Didn't Get from Kentucky Project," *Science*, 172 (April 30, 1971), pp. 458-460.

Health Service for American Indians, prepared by the Office of the Surgeon General, U. S. Department of Health, Education, and Welfare, Public Health Service Publication No. 531 (Washington, D.C.: U.S. Government Printing Office, 1957).

Health Service for American Indians, Appendix C, Report II, pp. 264-269.

Hearings Before the Subcommittee on Employment, Manpower and Poverty of the Committee on Labor and Public Welfare, United States Senate, Ninetieth Congress, July 11 and 12, 1967 (Washington, D.C.: U.S. Government Printing Office).

Hearings Before the Subcommittee on Health of the Elderly of the Special Committee on Aging, Costs and Delivery of Health Services to Older Americans, United States Senate, Ninetieth Congress, First Session, Part I (Washington, D.C.: U.S. Government Printing Office, 1967).

Hearings Before the Subcommittee on Medicare-Medicaid, Committee on Finance, United States Senate, Ninety-first Congress, Part 2, April 14, 15,

May 26, 27, June 2, 3, 15, 16, 1970 (Washington, D.C.: U.S. Government Printing Office, 1970).

Hearings Before the Select Committee on Nutrition and Human Needs of the United States Senate, Ninetieth Congress, Second Session, and Ninety-first Congress, Part 5B, Florida, Appendix (Washington, D.C.: U.S. Government Printing Office, 1969), p. 1835.

Heilbroner, R. L. "Benign Neglect in the United States," *TransAction* 7, No. 12 (October, 1970), pp. 15-22.

Hendin, H. *Black Suicide* (New York: Basic Books, 1969).

Herskovits, M. J. *The Myth of the Negro Past* (Boston: Beacon Press, 1941).

Herskovits, M. J. *The New World Negro*, edited by F. S. Herskovits (Bloomington: Indiana University Press, 1966).

Heston, L. L. "The Genetics of Schizophrenia and Schizoid Disease," *Science*, 167 (January 1970), pp. 249-256.

Hill, L. M., Sacramento Area Director, Bureau of Indian Affairs, as reported in the *Progress Report to the Legislature by the Senate Interim Committee on Indian Affairs* (Sacramento: California State Senate, 1955), pp. 241-242, 407-408.

Hochstim, J. R., Athanasopoulos, D. A., and Larkins, J. H. "Poverty Area Under the Microscope," *American Journal of Public Health*, 58 (October 1968), pp. 1815-1827.

Hollingshead, A. B., and Redlich, F. C. *Social Class and Mental Illness* (New York: John Wiley & Sons, 1958).

Hollingshead, A. B., and Redlich, F. C. "Social Stratification and Psychiatric Disorders," *American Sociological Review*, 18 (April 1953), pp. 163-169.

Howard, J., and Holman, B. L. "The Effects of Race and Occupation on Hypertension Mortality," *Milbank Memorial Fund Quarterly*, 48 (July 1970), pp. 263-296.

Hunger, U.S.A.: A Report by the Citizens' Board of Inquiry into Hunger and Malnutrition in the United States (Boston: Beacon Press, 1968), p. 11.

Hyde, R. W. "Socio-economic Aspects of Dental Caries," *New England Journal of Medicine*, 230 (1944), pp. 506-510.

"The Impact of Title VI on Health Facilities," *The George Washington Law Review*, 36 (May 1968), pp. 980-993.

Indian Health Service. *Suicide Among the American Indians*, U.S. Public Health Service Publication No. 1903 (Washington, D.C.: U.S. Government Printing Office, 1967).

Indian Health Service. *To the First Americans: The Third Annual Report on the Indian Health Program of the U.S. Public Health Service* (Washington, D.C.: U.S. Government Printing Office, 1969), p. 13.

Indian Health Services. *Trends and Services, 1969 Edition*, U.S. Department of Health, Education, and Welfare (Washington, D.C.: U.S. Government Printing Office, 1969) p. 8.

Ingham, J. M. "On Mexican Folk Medicine," *American Anthropologist*, 72 (February 1970), pp. 76-87.

Irelan, L. M. *Low Income Life Styles*, U.S. Department of Health, Education, and Welfare (Washington, D.C.: U.S. Government Printing Office, 1967).

Jackson, H. M. H. *A Century of Dishonor*, new edition, edited by Andrew F. Rolle, (reprinted, New York: Harper & Row, 1965).

Jaco, E. G. "Mental Health of the Spanish-American in Texas," in *Culture and Mental Health: Cross Cultural Studies*, edited by Marvin Opler (New York: The Macmillan Company, 1959), pp. 467-485.

Jaco, E. G., editor. *Patients, Physicians and Illness* (Glencoe, Ill.: The Free Press, 1958).

James, G. "Poverty and Public Health—New Outlooks: 1. Poverty as an Obstacle to Health Progress in Our Cities," *American Journal of Public Health*, 55 (November 1965), pp. 1757-1771.

Jensen, A. R. "How Much Can We Boost I. Q. and Scholastic Achievement?" *Harvard Educational Review*, 39 (Winter 1969), pp. 1-123.

Jewell, D. P. "A Case of a 'Psychotic Navaho Indian Male,'" in *Social Interaction and Patient Care*, edited by J. K. Skipper and R. C. Leonard (Philadelphia: Lippincott, 1965).

Johnson, C. A. "Nursing and Mexican American Folk Medicine," *Nursing Forum*, 3, No. 2 (1964), pp. 100-112.

Johnston, H. L. "A Smoother Road for Migrants," *American Journal of Nursing*, 66 (August 1966), pp. 1752-1756.

Jones, M. A. *American Immigration* (Chicago: University of Chicago Press, 1960).

Josephy, A. M., Jr. *The Indian Heritage of America* (New York: Alfred A. Knopf, 1969).

Kelly, C. H. "Fighting Poverty in Urban Areas" and "Fighting Poverty in Rural Areas," in *New Directions for Nurses*, edited by Bonnie and Vern Bullough (New York: Springer, 1971), pp. 248-259, 259-266.

Kelly, C. "Health Care in the Mississippi Delta," *American Journal of Nursing*, 69 (April 1969), pp. 759-763.

Kent, F. B. "Latin America Losing Much Needed Doctors," *Los Angeles Times*, September 17, 1971.

Kerner, O., Chairman, *Report of the National Advisory Commission on Civil Disorders* (Washington, D.C.: U.S. Government Printing Office, 1968).

Kiev, A. *Curanderismo: Mexican American Folk Psychiatry* (New York: The Free Press, 1968).

Kluckhohn, F. *Variations in Value Orientations* (Evanston, Ill.: Row, Peterson, 1961).

Knoch, H., Pasamanick, R., Harper, P. A., and Rider, R. "The Effect of Prematurity on Health and Growth," *American Journal of Public Health*, 49 (1959), pp. 1164-1173.

Koos, E. L. *The Health of Regionville* (New York: Columbia University Press, 1954).

Kosa, J., Antonovsky, A., and Zola, I. K., editors. *Poverty and Health: A Sociological Analysis* (Cambridge, Mass.: Commonwealth Fund Book, Harvard University Press, 1969).

Kotz, N. *Let Them Eat Promises: The Politics of Hunger in America* (New York: Anchor Books, 1971).

Kraus, B. S., with the collaboration of Jones, B. M. *Indian Health in Arizona* (Tucson: University of Arizona Press, 1954).

Kriesberg, L. *Mothers in Poverty: A Study of Fatherless Families* (Chicago: Aldine, 1970).

Kurth, A. *Children and Youth of Domestic Agricultural Migrant Families.* A survey paper reprinted from "Children and Youth in the 1960's," with permission of the 1960 White House Conference on Children and Youth (Washington, D.C.: U.S. Department of Health, Education, and Welfare, 1965).

Labovits, S. "Variation in Suicide Rates," in *Suicide*, edited by Jack P. Gibbs (New York: Harper & Row, 1968), pp. 57-73.

LaPouse, R., Monk, M. A., and Terris, M. "The Drift Hypothesis and Socio-Economic Differentials in Schizophrenia," *American Journal of Public Health*, 46 (August 1956), pp. 978-986.

Lepper, M. H., Lashof, J. C., Lerner, M., German, J., and Andeleman, S. L. "Approaches to Meeting Health Needs of Large Poverty Populations," *American Journal of Public Health*, 57 (July 1967), pp. 1153-1157.

Lewis, O. *La Vida: A Puerto Rican Family in the Culture of Poverty* (New York: Random House, 1965).

Lewis, O. *The Children of Sanchez* (New York: Vintage Books, 1961).

Lewis, O. "The Culture of Poverty," *Scientific American* (October 1966), pp. 19-25.

Lincoln, C. E. *The Negro Pilgrimage in America* (New York: Bantam Books, 1967).

Linden, G. "The Influence of Social Class in the Survival of Cancer Patients," *American Journal of Public Health*, 59 (February 1969), pp. 267-274.

Lindesmith, A. R. *Addiction and Opiates* (Chicago: Aldine, 1968).

Lindesmith, A. R. "Basic Problems in the Social Psychology of Addiction and a Theory," in *Narcotic Addiction*, edited by John A. O'Donnell and John C. Ball (New York: Harper & Row, 1966), pp. 91-109.

Lindsay, J. R., and Johnston, H. L. "Health Programs for Migrant Workers," excerpts from the proceedings of the 18th National Conference on Rural Health, 1965, Miami Beach, Florida, reprinted by the U.S. Department of Health, Education, and Welfare, 1966.

Liston, R. A. *The American Poor: A Report on Poverty in the United States* (New York: Dell, 1970).

Locke, B. Z., and Duvall, H. J. "Alcoholism Among First Admissions to Ohio Public Mental Hospitals," *Quarterly Journal of Studies*, 25 (1964), pp. 521-534.

Loughlin, B. W. "Pregnancy in the Navajo Culture," *Nursing Outlook*, 13 (March 1965), pp. 55-58.

Maddox, G. L. "Drinking Among Negroes: Inferences from the Drinking Patterns of Selected Negro Male Collegians," *Journal of Health and Social Behavior*, 8 (June 1967), pp. 114-120.

Maris, R. W. *Social Forces in Urban Suicide* (Homewood, Ill.: The Dorsey Press, 1969).

Martinez, C., and Martin, H. W. "Folk Diseases Among Urban Mexican-Americans," *Journal of the American Medical Association*, 196 (April 11, 1966), pp. 147-150.

Marx, G. T. *Protest and Prejudice: A Study of Belief in the Black Community* (New York: Harper & Row, 1967).

McBroom, W. H. "Illness, Behavior and Socioeconomic Status," *Journal of Health and Social Behavior*, 11 (December 1970), pp. 319-326.

McWilliams, C. *North from Mexico: The Spanish-Speaking People of the United States* (reprinted, New York: Greenwood Press, 1968).

Mechanic, D. "Correlates of Frustration Among British General Practitioners," *Journal of Health and Social Behavior*, 11 (June 1970), pp. 87-104.

Mechanic, D. *Mental Health and Social Policy* (Englewood Cliffs, N.J.: Prentice-Hall, 1969).

Mechanic, D. "The English National Health Service: Some Comparisons with the United States," *Journal of Health and Social Behavior*, 12 (March 1971), pp. 18-29.

Menninger, K. A. *Man Against Himself* (New York: Harcourt, Brace & Company, 1938).

Merton, R. K. "Social Structure and Anomie," *Social Theory and Social Structure* (Glencoe, Ill.: The Free Press, 1957), pp. 131-160.

Milio, N. *9226 Kercheval: The Storefront That Did Not Burn* (Ann Arbor: The University of Michigan Press, 1970).

Milio, N. "Values, Social Class and Community Health Services," *Nursing Research*, 16 (Winter 1967), pp. 26-31.

Milt, H., editor. *Health Care Problems of the Inner City: Report of the 1969 National Health Forum* (New York: 1969).

Morais, H. M. *The History of the Negro in Medicine* (New York: Publishers Company, 1968).

Morris, N. M., Hatch, M. H., and Chipman, S. S. "Alienation as a Deterrent to Well-Child Supervision," *American Journal of Public Health*, 56 (November 1966), pp. 1874-1882.

Moustafa, A. T., and Weiss, G. *Health Status and Practices of Mexican Americans*, Mexican-American Study Project, Advance Report II (Los Angeles: University of California, 1968).

Moynihan, D. P. *Maximum Feasible Misunderstanding: Community Action in the War on Poverty* (New York: The Free Press, 1969).

Munoz, R. *Nursing in the North 1867-1967* (The Alaska Nurses' Association, 1967).

Murphy, P. R. "Tuberculosis Control in San Francisco's Chinatown," *American Journal of Nursing*, 70 (May 1970), pp. 1044-1046.

Myers, J. K., and Bean, L. L., in collaboration with Pepper, M. P. *A Decade Later: A Follow-Up of Social Class and Mental Illness* (New York: John Wiley & Sons, 1968).

Myers, J. K., Bean, L. L., and Pepper, M. P. "Social Class and Psychiatric Disorders: A Ten Year Follow Up," *Journal of Health and Human Behavior*, 6 (Summer 1965), pp. 74-78.

Myers, J. K., and Roberts, B. N. *Family and Class Dynamics in Mental Illness* (New York: John Wiley & Sons, 1959).

Myrdal, G., with the assistance of Sterner, R., and Rose, A. *An American Dilemma: The Negro Problem and Modern Democracy* (New York: Harper & Brothers, 1944).

Nakagawa, H. "Family Health Care Patterns and Anomie," an unpublished Ph.D. dissertation, University of California at Los Angeles, 1968.

Nall, F. C., II, and Speilberg, J. "Social and Cultural Factors in the Responses of Mexican-Americans to Medical Treatment," *Journal of Health and Social Behavior*, 8 (December 1967), pp. 299-308.

Nash, R. M. "Compliance of Hospitals and Health Agencies with Title VI of the Civil Rights Act," *American Journal of Public Health*, 58 (February 1968), pp. 246-251.

Nash, R. M. "Integration in Health Facilities," *American Journal of Nursing*, 66 (November 1966), pp. 2480-2482.

National Center for Health Statistics. *Differentials in Health Characteristics by Color, United States, July 1965-June 1967*, U.S. Department of Health, Education, and Welfare, Public Health Service Publication No. 1000, Series 10, No. 56 (Washington, D.C.: U.S. Government Printing Office, 1969).

National Center for Health Statistics. *Medical Care, Health Status and Family Income*, Vital and Health Statistics, U.S. Department of Health, Education, and Welfare, Public Health Service Publication No. 1000, Series 10, No. 9 (Washington, D.C.: U.S. Government Printing Office, 1964), p. 6.

National Center for Health Statistics. *Selected Dental Findings in Adults by Age, Race and Sex, United States, 1960-1962*, U.S. Department of Health, Education, and Welfare, Public Health Service Publication No. 1000, Series 11, No. 7 (Washington, D.C.: U.S. Government Printing Office, 1965).

National Center for Health Statistics. *Three Views of Hypertension and Heart Disease*, U.S. Department of Health, Education, and Welfare, Public Health Service Publication No. 1000, Series 2, No. 22 (Washington, D.C.: U.S. Government Printing Office, 1967).

National Institute of Mental Health and the Indian Health Service. *Suicide Among the American Indians*, Public Health Service Publication No. 1903 (Washington, D.C.: U.S. Government Printing Office, 1967).

Norman, J. C. *Medicine in the Ghetto* (New York: Appleton-Century-Crofts, 1969).

O'Donnell, J. A., and Ball, J. C., editors. *Narcotic Addiction* (New York: Harper & Row, 1966).

Opler, M. K. *Culture and Mental Health* (New York: The Macmillan Company, 1959).

Orshansky, M. "The Poverty Roster," *Sources* (Chicago: The Blue Cross Association, 1968), pp. 4-19.

Orshansky, M. "Who Was Poor in 1966?" *Research and Statistics Note*, No. 23 (Washington, D.C.: U.S. Department of Health, Education, and Welfare, 1967), Table 6.

Otterbein, K. F. "Caribbean Family Organization: A Comparative Analysis," *American Anthropologist*, 67 (February 1965), pp. 66-79.

Pasamanick, B. "A Survey of Mental Disease in an Urban Population," in *Mental Health and Segregation*, edited by Martin M. Grossack (New York: Springer, 1963), pp. 150-157.

Pelton, W. J., Dunbar, J. B., McMillan, R. S., Moller, P., and Wolff, A. E. *The Epidemiology of Oral Health* (Cambridge, Mass.: Harvard University Press, 1969).

Pettigrew, T. F. *A Profile of the Negro American* (Princeton, N.J.: D. Van Nostrand, 1964).

Pilisak, M., and Pilisak, P., editors. *Poor Americans: How the Poor White Live* (Chicago: Aldine, 1971).

Piven, F. F., and Cloward, R. A. "The Relief of Welfare," *Transaction*, 8 (May 1971), pp. 31-39, 52-53.

Proshansky, H., and Newton, P. "The Nature and Meaning of Negro Self-Identity," in *Social Class, Race and Psychological Development*, edited by M. Deutsch, I. Katz, and A. Jensen (New York: Holt, Rinehart & Winston, 1968), pp. 178-218.

Puckett, N. N. *Folk Beliefs of the Southern Negro* (reprinted, New York: Dover, 1969).

Rainwater, L. *And the Poor Get Children* (Chicago: Quadrangle Books, 1960).

Rainwater, L. *Behind Ghetto Walls* (Chicago: Aldine, 1970).

Rainwater, L., and Yancey, W. L. *The Moynihan Report and the Politics of Controversy* (Cambridge, Mass.: The M.I.T. Press, 1967).

Randolph, V. *Ozark Magic and Folklore* (New York: Dover, 1947).

Rehabilitating the Narcotic Addict, U.S. Department of Health, Education, and Welfare, Report of Institute on New Developments in the Rehabilitation of the Narcotic Addict, Forth Worth, Texas, February 16-18, 1966 (Washington, D.C.: U.S. Government Printing Office, 1966).

Reitzes, D. C. *Negroes and Medicine* (Cambridge, Mass.: Commonwealth Fund Study, Harvard University Press, 1958).

Richard, M. P. "The Negro Physician: Babbitt or Revolutionary," *Journal of Health and Social Behavior*, 10 (December 1969), pp. 265-274.

Riessman, F. *Strategies Against Poverty* (New York: Random House, 1969).

Riis, J. A. *How the Other Half Lives* [1890] (reprinted; New York: Sagamore Press, 1957).

Roach, J. L., Lewis, L. S., and Beauchamp, M. A. "The Effects of Race and Socio-Economic Status on Family Planning," *Journal of Health and Social Behavior*, 4 (March 1963), pp. 40-45.

Robertson, H. R. "Removing Barriers to Health Care," *Nursing Outlook*, 17 (September 1969), pp. 43-46.

Robins, L. N. "Social Correlates of Psychiatric Disorders," *Journal of Health and Social Behavior*, 10 (June 1969), pp. 95-104.

Robins, L. N., and Murphy, G. E. "Drug Use in a Normal Population of Young Negro Men," *American Journal of Public Health*, 57 (September 1967), pp. 1580-1596.

Roemer, M. I. "Health Care—Financing and Delivery Around the World," *American Journal of Nursing*, 71 (June 1971), pp. 1158-1163.

Roemer, M. I. "Health Resources and Services in the Watts Area of Los Angeles," *California's Health* (February-March 1966), pp. 123-143.

Roemer, M. I. "Highlights of Soviet Health Services," *Milbank Memorial Fund Quarterly*, 15, No. 4 (October 1962), pp. 381-385.

Roemer, M. I. *The Organization of Medical Care Under Social Security* (Geneva: International Labour Office, 1969).

Rosen, G. *A History of Public Health* (New York: M.D. Publications, 1958).

Rosenthal, R., and Jacobson, L. *Pygmalion in the Classroom: Teacher Expectation and Pupils' Intellectual Development* (New York: Holt, Rinehart & Winston, 1969).

Rosenthal, R., and Jacobson, L. "Self Fulfilling Prophesies in the Classroom: Teacher's Expectations as Unintended Determinants of Pupils' Intellectual Competence," in *Social Class, Race and Psychological Development*, edited by M. Deutsch, I. Katz, and A. Jensen (New York: Holt, Rinehart & Winston, 1968), pp. 219-253.

Rowden, D. W., Michel, J. B., Dillehay, R. C., and Martin, H. W. "Judgements About Candidates for Psychotherapy: The Influence of Social Class and Insight-Verbal Ability," *Journal of Health and Social Behavior*, 11 (March 1970), pp. 51-58.

Rubel, A. J. *Across the Tracks: Mexican-Americans in a Texas City* (Austin: University of Texas Press, 1966).

Samora, J., editor. *La Raza: Forgotten Americans* (Notre Dame, Ind.: University of Notre Dame Press, 1966).

Sandifer, M. G., Jr. "Social Psychiatry a Hundred Years Ago," *American Journal of Psychiatry*, 188 (February 1962), pp. 749-750.

Saunders, L. *Cultural Differences and Medical Care: The Case of the Spanish-Speaking People of the Southwest* (New York: Russell Sage Foundation, 1954).

Scheinfeldt, J. "Opening Doors Wider in Nursing," *American Journal of Nursing*, 67 (July 1967), pp. 1461-1464.

Schmidt, W., Smart, R. G., and Moss, M. K. *Social Class and the Treatment of Alcoholism: An Investigation of Social Class as a Determinant of Diagnoses, Prognosis and Therapy* Brookside Monograph for the Addiction Research Foundation, No. 7, (Toronto: University of Toronto Press, 1968).

Schorr, A. L. "The Case for Federal Welfare," *The Nation* (May 3, 1971), pp. 5551-5557.

Schulman, S., and Smith, A. M. "The Concept of 'Health' Among Spanish Speaking Villagers of New Mexico and Colorado," *Journal of Health and Human Behavior*, 4 (Winter 1963), pp. 226-234.

Schulz, V. E., and Schwab, E. H. "Arteriolar Hypertension in the American Negro," *American Heart Journal*, 11 (January 1936), pp. 66-74.

Schwarzweller, H. K., Brown, J. S., and Mangalem, J. J. *Mountain Families in Transition* (University Park: Pennsylvania State University Press, 1971).

Seham, M. "Discrimination Against Negroes in Hospitals," *New England Journal of Medicine*, 271 (October 29, 1964), pp. 940-943.

Senior, C. *Our Citizens from the Caribbean* (New York: McGraw-Hill, 1965).

Senior, C. *The Puerto Ricans* (Chicago: Quadrangle Books, 1965).

Shapiro, S., Schlesinger, E. R., and Nesbitt, R. E. L., Jr. *Infant, Perinatal, Maternal and Childhood Mortality in the United States* (Cambridge: Harvard University Press, 1968).

Shelton, E. "Prejudices Hit Women in Medicine," *Los Angeles Times,* October 4, 1970.

Simmons, O. G. "Implications of Social Class for Public Health," in *A Sociological Framework for Patient Care,* edited by Jeanette R. Rolta and Edith S. Deck (New York: John Wiley & Sons, 1966).

Social Security Administration. *The Evolution of Medicare: From Idea to Law,* Research Report, No. 29 (Washington, D.C.: U.S. Government Printing Office, 1969), pp. 5-16.

Sobey, F. *The Nonprofessional Revolution in Mental Health* (New York: Columbia University Press, 1970).

Somers, H. M., and Somers, A. R. *Doctors, Patients and Health Insurance: The Organization and Financing of Medical Care* (Washington, D.C.: The Brookings Institution, 1961).

Sources: A Blue Cross Report on Health Problems of the Poor (Chicago: The Blue Cross Association, 1968).

Srole, L., Langner, T. S., Michael, S. T., Opler, M. K., and Rennie, T. C. *Mental Health in the Metropolis: The Midtown Manhattan Study,* Vol. 1 (New York: McGraw-Hill, 1962).

Stamler, J., and Stamler, R. "Psychological Factors and Hypertension Disease in Low-Income Middle Aged Negro Men in Chicago," *Circulation,* 26 (October 1962) Part 2, p. 790.

Stanley, J. C. "Predicting College Success of the Educationally Disadvantaged," *Science,* 171 (February 1971), pp. 640-646.

Star, J. "Cook County Hospital: The Terrible Place," *Look* (May 18, 1971), pp. 24-33.

Storlie, F. *Nursing and the Social Conscience* (New York: Appleton-Century-Crofts, 1970).

Strickland, S. P. "Can Slum Children Learn?" *American Education,* 7 (July 1971), pp. 3-7.

Suchman, E. A. *Sociology and the Field of Public Health* (New York: Russell Sage Foundation, 1963).

Suicide Among the American Indians: Two Workshops, Aberdeen, South Dakota, September, 1967, Lewistown, Montana, November, 1967, U.S. Department of Health, Education, and Welfare, Public Health Service Publication No. 1903 (Washington, D.C.: U.S. Government Printing Office, 1969).

Suttles, G. D. *The Social Order of the Slum: Ethnicity and Territory in the Inner City* (Chicago: University of Chicago Press, 1968).

Taeuber, K. E., and Taeuber, A. F. *Negroes in Cities* (Chicago: Aldine, 1965).

Tao-Kim-Nai, A. M. "Orientals are Stoic," in *Social Interaction and Patient Care,* edited by J. Skipper and R. C. Leonard (Philadelphia: Lippincott, 1965).

Terris, M., and Gold, E. M. "An Epidemiologic Study of Prematurity," *American Journal of Obstetrics and Gynecology,* 103 (February 1, 1969), pp. 371-379.

"The People Left Behind: The Rural Poor, A Report by the President's Commission on Rural Poverty," in *Poverty in America*, edited by L. A. Ferman, J. L. Kornblugh, and A. Haber (Ann Arbor: University of Michigan Press, revised edition, 1968), pp. 152-153.

The Social Psychology of George Herbert Mead, edited by A. Strauss (Chicago: University of Chicago Press, 1956).

Their Daily Bread: A Study of the National School Lunch Program (New York: Committee on School Lunch Participation, 1968).

"Those Amazing Cuban Emigres," *Fortune*, 74 (October 1966), pp. 144-149.

Tompkins, D. C. *Drug Addiction: A Bibliography* (Berkeley: Bureau of Public Administration, University of California, 1960).

Townsend, J. G. "Indian Health—Past, Present, and Future," in *The Changing Indian*, edited by O. LaFarge (Norman: University of Oklahoma Press, 1942), pp. 28-41.

Tunley, R. *The American Health Scandal* (New York: Harper & Row, 1966).

Turner, J. R. "Social Mobility and Schizophrenia," *Journal of Health and Social Behavior*, 9 (September 1968), pp. 194-203.

Tuttle, W. M., Jr. *Race Riot* (New York: Atheneum, 1970).

Udry, J. R., Bauman, K. E., Morris, N. M., and Chase, C. L. "Social Class, Social Mobility, and Prematurity: A Test of the Childhood Environment Hypothesis for Negro Women," *Journal of Health and Social Behavior*, 11 (September 1970), pp. 190-195.

United Nations, Statistical Office. *Statistical Yearbook, 1968* (New York: United Nations Publishing Service, 1969), pp. 99-100.

United States Bureau of the Census. *Current Population Reports*, Series P-23, No. 28, "Revision in Poverty Statistics, 1959-1968" (Washington, D.C.: U.S. Government Printing Office, 1969).

United States Bureau of the Census. *Current Population Reports*, Series F-60, No. 76, "24 Million Americans—Poverty in the United States, 1969" (Washington, D.C.: U.S. Government Printing Office, 1970).

United States Bureau of the Census. *Statistical Abstract of the United States, 1970* (Washington, D.C.: U.S. Government Printing Office, 1970), p. 39, Table 47.

United States Commission on Civil Rights. *Civil Rights '63* (Washington, D.C.: U.S. Government Printing Office, 1963), pp. 137-138.

United States Commission on Civil Rights, *Title VI . . . One Year After: A Survey of Desegregation of Health and Welfare Services in the South* (Washington, D.C.: U.S. Government Printing Office, 1966).

United States Department of Health, Education, and Welfare. *Health Services for American Indians* Public Health Service Publication No. 531 (Washington, D.C.: U.S. Government Printing Office, 1957).

United States Department of Health, Education, and Welfare, Public Health Service. *Human Investment Programs: Delivery of Health Services for the Poor*, December, 1967, 12 (Washington, D.C.: U.S. Government Printing Office, 1967).

United States Department of Health, Education, and Welfare, Indian Health Service, *Indian Health Services: Trends and Services, 1969 Edition* (Washington, D.C.: U.S. Government Printing Office, 1969).

United States Department of Health, Education, and Welfare, Public Health Service, *Nursing Careers Among the American Indians* (Washington, D.C.: U.S. Government Printing Office, 1970), p. 1.

United States Department of Health, Education, and Welfare. *The Impact of Medicare: An Annotated Bibliography of Selected Sources* (Washington, D.C.: U.S. Government Printing Office, 1969).

United States Department of Health, Education, and Welfare. *Variations in Birth Weight: Legitimate Live Births, United States, 1963*, Vital and Health Statistics, Public Health Service Publication No. 1000, Series 22, No. 8 (Washington, D.C.: U.S. Government Printing Office, 1964).

United States Department of Health, Education, and Welfare. *Vital Statistics of the United States*, Vol. II, *Mortality* (Washington, D.C.: U.S. Government Printing Office, 1968).

United States Department of Health, Education, and Welfare. *Volume of Physician Visits, United States, July, 1966–June, 1967*, Vital and Health Statistics (National Center for Health Statistics, Series 10, No. 49), p. 21.

United States Department of Labor. *The Negro Family: The Case for National Action* (Washington, D.C.: U.S. Government Printing Office, 1965).

United States Division of Indian Health. *Indians on Federal Reservation in the United States, Phoenix Area: Arizona, California, Nevada, Utah*, U.S. Department of Health, Education, and Welfare, Public Health Service Publication No. 615, Part 6 (January 1961), p. 32.

United States Division of Indian Health, Program Analysis and Special Studies Branch. *Eskimos, Indians, and Aleuts of Alaska—A Digest*, U.S. Department of Health, Education, and Welfare (Washington, D.C.: U.S. Government Printing Office, 1963).

"United States Government Expands Migrant Health Program," *American Journal of Nursing*, 68 (July 1968), pp. 1405-1406.

United States Social Security Administration, *Social Security Programs Throughout the World* (Washington, D.C.: U.S. Government Printing Office, 1967).

Valentine, C. A. *Culture and Poverty: Critique and Counter Proposals* (Chicago: University of Chicago Press, 1968).

Wakefield, D. *Island in the City: Puerto Ricans in New York* (New York: Corinth Books, 1960).

Wald, L. *The House on Henry Street* (New York: Henry Holt and Co., 1915).

Walsh, J. "Stanford School of Medicine (1) Problems over More than Money," *Science* (February 12, 1971), pp. 551-553.

Warne, F. J. *The Tide of Immigration* (New York: D. Appleton and Co., 1916).

Watkins, E. L. "Low-Income Negro Mothers—Their Decision to Seek Prenatal Care," *American Journal of Public Health*, 58 (April 1968), pp. 655-667.

"Watts: Everything Has Changed—and Nothing," *Newsweek* (August 24, 1970), pp. 58-60.

Watts, W. "Social Class, Ethnic Background and Patient Care," *Nursing Forum*, 6, No. 2 (1967).

Weiner, G., Rider, R. V., Oppel, W. C., and Harper, P. A. "Correlates of Low Birth Weight: Psychological Status at Eight to Ten Years of Age," *Pediatric Research*, 2 (March 1968), pp. 110-118.

Weiner, G., Rider, R. V., Oppel, W. C., Fischer, L., and Harper, P. A. "Correlates of Low Birth Weight: Psychological Status at Six to Seven Years of Age," *Pediatrics*, 35 (1965), pp. 434-444.

Weller, J. E. *Yesterday's People: Life in Contemporary Appalachia* (Lexington: University of Kentucky Press, 1965).

Westoff, C. F., Potter, R. C., Jr., and Sagi, P. C. *The Third Child* (Princeton: Princeton University Press, 1963).

Westoff, C. F., Potter, R. C., Jr., Sagi, P. C., and Mishler, E. *Family Growth in Metropolitan America* (Princeton: Princeton University Press, 1961).

Whelpton, P. K., and Kiser, C. V. *Social and Psychological Factors Affecting Fertility*, Vol. V (New York: Milbank Memorial Fund, 1958).

White House Conference on Food, Nutrition and Health, Final Report. Jean Mayer, chairman (Washington, D.C.: U.S. Government Printing Office, 1970).

Whiteman, M., and Deutsch, M. "Social Disadvantage as Related to Intellective and Language Development," in *Social Class, Race and Psychological Development*, edited by M. Deutsch, I. Katz, and A. R. Jensen (New York: Holt, Rinehart & Winston, 1968), pp. 86-114.

Willie, C. V. "The Social Class of Patients that Public Health Nurses Prefer to Serve," *American Journal of Public Health*, 50 (August 1960), pp. 1126-1136.

Wirth, L. *The Ghetto* (Chicago: University of Chicago Press, 1928).

Wirth, L. "The Problem of Minority Groups," in *The Science of Man in the World Crisis*, edited by Ralph Linton (New York: Columbia University Press, 1945), pp. 347-372.

Woodson, C. G. *The Negro Professional Man and the Community* (Johnson Reprint Co., 1934).

Yates, J. A. "Breakthrough in Minnesota," *American Journal of Nursing*, 70 (March 1970), pp. 563-565.

Yerby, A. S. "Health Departments, Hospitals and Health Services," mimeographed copy of an address given at the Fiftieth Anniversary Celebration, October 6, 1966, at The Johns Hopkins School of Hygiene and Public Health.

Yerby, A. S. "Improving Care for the Disadvantaged," *American Journal of Nursing*, 68 (May 1968), p. 1044.

Yost, E. *The U.S. Health Industry—The Costs of Acceptable Medical Care* (New York: Frederick A. Praeger, 1969).

Zborowski, M. *People in Pain* (San Francisco: Jossey-Bass, Inc., 1969).

Additional references

Coles, R. Migrants, Sharecroppers, Mountaineers, Vol II of *Children in Crisis* (Boston: Little Brown and Co, 1971).

Davis, M. M. Jr. *Immigrant Health and the Community* 1921 (Montclair, New Jersey: Patterson Smith Reprint Series, Reprinted, 1970).

Elling, R. H. *National Health Care: Issues and Problems in Socialized Medicine* (Chicago: Aldine-Atherton, 1971).

Freidson, E., and Lorber, J. eds. *Medical Men and Their Work: A Sociological Reader* (Chicago: Aldine-Atherton, 1971).

Hirshfield, D. S. *The Campaign for Compulsory Health Insurance in the United States from 1932 to 1943* (Cambridge, Mass: Harvard University Press, 1970).

Scrimshaw, N. S. and Gordon, J. E. *Malnutrition, Learning, and Behavior* (Cambridge, Mass: M.I.T. Press, 1971).

Index

Addams, Jane, 34, 35
Agriculture
  economic factors, 112
  effects of Depression, 111
  revolution in, 110-11
Alaskan natives, 99, 100, 101
Alcoholism, 142-43
American Indians. *See* Native Americans
  icans
Anemia, relation to poverty, 119-20
Anomie
  among native Americans, 102
  result of poverty, 56
  result of segregation, 139
Appalachia, 113-15
  economic conditions, 113-14
  geographic definition, 113
  migration from, 114-15
  population statistics, 113
Ataque, 84-85

Barbiturates, 143
Bilis, 84
Black Americans, 37-59. *See also*
  Discrimination; Slavery
  African cultural heritage, 41-42
  African family system, 41
  alcoholism among, 143
  and culture of poverty, 54-57
  dental care, 58-59
  early history, 39-41
  early leaders, 44-45
  educational level, 48
  folk medicine, 53-54

Black Americans (Cont.)
  health
    life expectancy, 47
    maternal mortality, 8, 58
    preventive care, 54-59
  health care. *See* Health care, black
    Americans
  health professionals, 151-53
    dentists, 152
    nurses, 152-53, 155
    physicians, 151-52
    recruitment, 153-54
  housing discrimination, 3-5
  income level, 49-50
  increasing militancy, 46
  job discrimination, 46, 48-49
  lynching of, 43
  migration to urbanized North,
    45-46
  race riots, 46, 140-41
  during Reconstruction, 43
  segregation
    and alienation, 57
    black medical schools, 151
    dental education, 152
    imposition of, 43
    medical education, 151-52
    nursing homes, 163
    redress by courts, 46
    reinforcement of negative self-
      image, 139
  self-image, 138
  trends within the community,
    44-46
    black power, 45

Black Americans (Cont.)
    gradualism (Washington), 44
    integration and equality (Du-Bois), 44, 45
    nationalism (Garvey), 45
Brain damage
  and malnutrition, 122-23
  and premature birth, 123
Brewster, Mary, 34
Bubonic plague, 1

Century of Dishonor, 93
Chinese-Americans, 22, 28-29
Citizen's Crusade Against Poverty, 119
Clay eating, 121-22
Collier, John, 96
Commodity distribution programs, 124-25
Contract labor, 40, 66-67
Cuba, economic relationship to United States
  before Castro, 72-73
  since Castro, 73
Cuban-Americans, 72-75
Cubans
  health problems, 74-75
  high socioeconomic status of recent refugees, 74
  immigration to United States
    before Castro, 73
    since Castro, 73-74
Culture of poverty. *See* Poverty, culture of
Curandero, 80-84, 86

Dawes General Allotment Act, 93-94
Dental care, relation to socioeconomic status, 58-59, 150
Dentistry
  changes in training, 150
  discrimination against women, 156
  proportion of blacks, 152
Discrimination. *See also* Black Americans, segregation
  against black Americans, 48, 52-53, 151-53, 157-63
  against Chinese-Americans, 28-29
  effect on mental health, 139-41

Discrimination (Cont.)
  in health care. *See* Health care, discrimination
  against immigrants, 19
  in medical education, 10, 105, 147-48, 151-52
    black Americans, 105
    Jews, 151
    native Americans, 105
    women, 156
Drug addiction
  causes, 143
  and socioeconomic status, 143
DuBois, W. E. B., 44-45

Empacho, 82
Epidemics, 19th-century America, 33-34
Ethnic groups. *See* Minority groups
Ethnic identity and poverty, 5
Ethnic neighborhoods, 24. *See also* Ghetto

Fair Employment Practice Acts, 46
Family planning and socioeconomic status, 56-57
Folk medicine
  black Americans, 53-54
    magical versus empirical beliefs, 53-54
    origins, 53-54
  Mexican-American, 79-84
    disease classification, 81-84
      dislocations of internal organs, 81, 83
      hot and cold imbalance, 81-82
      illnesses of emotional origin, 84
      illnesses of magical origin, 83-84
  Puerto Rican, 81, 84-85
Food stamp programs, 125

Geiger, H. Jack, 123-24
Germ theory, 33
Ghetto, 24, 26
Grapes of Wrath, 111

Hallucinogenic drugs, 143
Haymarket Riot, 29
Head Start program, 137
Health. *See also* Black Americans, health; Immigrants, health; Mexican-Americans, health; Puerto Ricans, health
  and ethnic status, 7
  and socioeconomic status, 7-12, 49-51
Health care. *See also* Public health
  black Americans, 47-59
  changing nature
    centralization in hospitals, 12, 149-60
    in child birth, 12-13
    in doctor-patient relationship, 167-68
    in nursing, 149-50
  charity, 50-51, 149
  discrimination, 5, 52-53, 82-83, 157-64
    in Chicago, 1950s, 158-59
    effect of Medicare, 162-64
    by hospitals, 82-83, 157-63
      Hill-Burton hospitals, 160-61
    in nursing homes, 163
    by physicians, 159
    prohibition by Supreme Court, 161
    resultant communication problems, 157
    role of federal government, 159-63
  fee-for-service commodity, 49-50, 148-49
  foreign-trained physicians, 155-56
  fragmentation, 11, 15-16
  Mexican-Americans, 76-77, 79-80, 85-86
    collaboration with folk practitioners, 85-86
    language barriers, 76-77
  native Americans, 97-106
    Alaskan natives, 99
    cooperation with medicine man, 105-6
    Indian Health Service facilities, 100
    native health workers, 105
    prior to 20th century, 97
    problem of trust, 105-6

Health care (Cont.)
    transfer to Public Health Service, 98-99
  need for comprehensive plan, 14-16
  preventive, 11, 54-59
    and socioeconomic status, 54-59
  scientific breakthroughs, 13
Health insurance, voluntary, 13, 50
  influence on health care, 13
Henry Street Settlement, 34
Hill-Burton Act, 52, 160-61
Hospital Survey and Construction Act. *See* Hill-Burton Act
Hull House, 34
Hunger. *See* Malnutrition

Immigrants, 18-35
  Amish, Old Order, 23
  assimilation, 19, 22-23
  Chinese, 22, 28-29
    exclusion, 28-29
  community health services, 34-35
  discrimination, 19, 25-27
  Dutch, 25
  18th-century, 23-24
  emigration to homelands, 22-23
  exploitation of, 25
  French Huguenot, 23
  after French Revolution, 23
  German-speaking, 23
  health, 30-35
    effects of sea voyage, 30-31
    epidemics, 33-34
    health care, 34
  Irish, 25-26
  Jewish, 26-27
  living conditions, 32-33
  Mennonite, 23
  Mormon, 23, 28, 32
  after Napoleon Wars, 23
  19th-century, 21-24
  Orthodox Christian, 26
  patterns of settlement, 24, 31-32
  problems of adjustment, 19
  and racism, 27-29
  Roman Catholic, 25-26
  Scotch-Irish, 23
  Swedish, 23

Immigration controls, 27-30
  literacy tests, 29
  restrictive quotas, 29-30
Immigration Restrictive League, 28
Indian Reorganization Act, 96
Indians, American. *See* Native Americans
Infant mortality rate
  factors influencing, 9-10
  of native Americans, 100, 101, 104
  and socioeconomic status, 8-10
  of United States versus other countries, 8-10
Intelligence
  environmental determinants, 136
  genetic determinants, 136

Jackson, Helen Hunt, 93
Jensen, Arthur, 136
Jim Crow legislation, 43

King, Martin Luther, Jr., 46
King Philip's War, 92
Knights of the White Camelia, 42
Ku-Klux Klan, 42
Kwashiorkor
  among native Americans, 120
  and poverty, 120-21

Laundry starch eating, 121-22
Life expectancy
  native Americans, 100
  whites versus nonwhites, 8

Mal aire, 83-84
Mal ojo, 83-84
Malnutrition, 117-26
  and brain damage, 122-23
  clay and laundry starch eating, 121-22
  and inadequate nutritional knowledge, 121
  among migrant workers, 122
  in Mississippi, 118-19
  and premature births, 123
  among Puerto Ricans, 78
  Senate investigation, 118-119

Malnutrition (Cont.)
  solutions, 123-26. *See also* Com-distribution programs; Food stamp programs; Mound Bayou Clinic; School lunch programs lunch programs
  effectiveness, 126
Marasmus
  among native Americans, 120
  and poverty, 120-21
Marijuana, 143
Maternal mortality rate, 8, 58
Mather, Increase, 92
Medical care. *See* Health care
Medical education
  changes in, 13, 149-50
  discrimination. *See* Discrimination in medical education
  elitist nature, 147-48
  recruitment of minority candidates, 153-54
  need for compensatory education, 154
Medicare, effect on hospital integration, 52-53, 162-64
Medicine. *See* Health care
Medicine man, Indian, 97, 105, 106
Mental health. *See also* Mental illness
  effects of discrimination, 139-41
  anger, 140-41
  effects of poverty on children, 135-39
  effects of segregation, 139
Mental illness. *See also* Mental health
  biological determinants, 132
  environmental determinants, 132
  and ethnic identity, 134-35
  hospital care, 133
  coping mechanisms, 133
  importance of early diagnosis, 7-8
  psychiatric versus sociological view, 132
  and socioeconomic status, 7-8, 129-44
  complexity of relationship, 130-32
  empirical studies, 130
  ethnocentricity of therapists, 133-34
  relative distribution of diagnoses, 130-31

Mental illness (Cont.)
    relative distribution of disorders, 131-32
    schizophrenia, 129-30
    type of treatment recieved, 132-34
Meriam, Lewis, 96
Mexican-Americans, 63-70, 75-77, 79-86
  conferral of citizenship, 64
  contract laborers, World War I period, 66-67
  cultural continuity with Mexicans, 66
  cultural heritage, 69-70
  discrimination against, 69
  economic contributions, 65-66
  emigration to Mexico during Depression, 67
  folk medicine. *See* Folk medicine, Mexican-American
  health, 75-77
    differential mortality rates, 75-76
    poverty-related problems, 75
  health care. *See* Health care, Mexican-Americans
  housing patterns, 69
  immigration to United States, 65-68
  labor source, World War II and after, 68
  patterns of settlement, 66
  population distribution, 68-69
  racial origins, 64-65
  recruitment in nursing education, 154
  representation among health professionals, 155
  stereotype, 70
Mexican-American War, 64
Migrant workers, 115-16, 125
  living conditions, 116
  malnutrition among, 122
  noncoverage by labor statutes, 116
  patterns of migration, 115-16
  population, 115
  socioeconomic difficulties, 116
  working conditions, 116
Migration
  of black Americans, 45-46

Migration (Cont.)
  effects on Puerto Rican health, 78-79
  farm to city, 37-38, 111
  South to North and West, 38, 45-46
Minorities
  American. *See* Black Americans; Native Americans; Immigrants
  classification, 20
  created by European imperialism, 21
  defined, 2
  in Europe, 20-21
  negative self-image, 138-39
  protection by constitutional guarantees, 18
  in South Africa and Rhodesia, 21
  Spanish-speaking. *See* Cuban-Americans; Mexican-Americans; Puerto Ricans
Mollera ciada, 83
Mound Bayou Clinic, 123-24

Narcotics, 143
National Advisory Commission on Civil Disorders, 141
National Association of Colored People, 45
National Medical Association, 159
National Urban League, 45
Native Americans, 89-106
  anomie, 102
  attempts to assimilate, 93-95, 96
  classification, 89-90
  conferral of citizenship, 95-96
  cultural integrity versus assimilation, 96-97
  discrimination against, in medical education, 105
  education, 94-95
  government policy
    after King Philip's War, 92-93
    changes during 19th century, 93-94
    Dawes General Allotment Act, 93-94
    Snyder Act, 94-95
    support of tribal integrity, 96

Native Americans (Cont.)
    Wheeler Howard Act, 96
   health, 97-98, 100-4
    alcoholism, 100, 102-3
    effects of poverty, 104
    fatal accidents, 100, 101
    infant mortality, 100, 101, 104
    kwashiorkor, 120
    life expectancy, 100
    marasmus, 120
    mortality rates, 101
    recent improvements, 100
    suicide rate, 100, 101
    trachoma, 97-98
    tuberculosis, 101, 103-4
   health care. *See* Health care, native
    Americans
   health professionals, 155
   hostility toward, 95-96
   impact of European settlement,
    91-92
    disease, 92
    the horse, 91
    metal tools, 91
    new political alliances, 91-92
    weapons, 91
   misunderstanding of, 94-95
   population distribution, 90
   precolonial, 90-91
    cultural variation, 91
    physical variation, 91
   removal to West, 93
   voting rights, 95-96
Near-poor, 6, 48
Negroes. *See* Black Americans
New York City Metropolitan Board
   of Health, 33
Niagara Movement, 44-45
Nino, Pedro Alonzo, 39
Nursing
   changes during 20th century,
    13-14
   discrimination against men, 156
   professionalization, 148
   proportion of Blacks, 152
Nursing education
   admission of blacks, 152-53
   recruitment of minority candi-
    dates, 154-55

Oakies, 38, 111
Opening the Doors Wider in Nursing
   (ODWIN), 155
Organic Act, 70

Parasitic diseases, among Puerto Ricans, 78
Partera, 80-81
Pasteur, Louis, 33
Pequot War, 92
Pharmacy, 148, 150
Point Du Sable, Jean Baptiste, 39
Poliomyelitis
   research and therapy programs, 15
   socioeconomic distribution, 14-15
Poor Americans. *See* Poverty; Socioeconomic status
Poverty
   acute versus chronic, 55
   causes, 109-10
   culture of, 54-57
    alienation, 56
    characteristics, 55-56
   distribution
    by age, 6, 110
    among minorities, 6
   and the elderly, 110
   and ethnic identity, 5, 109
   and health, 7-12, 117-26
    infant anemia, 119-20
    kwashiorkor, 120
    marasmus, 120
   and health care, 10-11, 148-49
   and housing, 2-4
   incidence, 6, 47-48, 117
   indices of, 5-6
    Social Security Administration
    index, 5-6, 47, 117
   and malnutrition, 117-26. *See
    also* Malnutrition
   measurement of, 5-6
   and mental development. *See* So-
    cioeconomic status and men-
    tal development
   and mental illness. *See* Mental ill-
    ness and socioeconomic sta-
    tus

Poverty (Cont.)
and negative self-image, 138-39
resulting from technological
change, 110
rural, 110-16
displacement of farm families,
111-12
effects of agricultural revolution,
110-11
elimination of farms, 111-12
family size, 112
migrant workers. See Migrant
workers
and white Americans, 109-10
Premature birth
and brain damage, 123
and malnutrition, 123
and socioeconomic status, 123
Preventive health care. See Health
care, preventive
Public health programs, 14-15
bias toward needs of upper and
middle classes, 14-15
for poliomyelitis, 14-15
for tuberculosis, 15
Puerto Ricans, 70-72, 77-79, 81,
84-85
acquisition of American citizenship, 70
folk medicine. See Folk medicine,
Puerto Rican
health, 77-79
effect of migration, 78-79
malnutrition, 78
parasitic diseases, 78
rat bites, 77
tuberculosis, 77-78
health professionals, 155
migration to United States, 71
racial origins, 71-72
socioeconomic status, 72
Puerto Rico, 70-71
acquisition by United States, 70
impact on health, 71
impact on population growth, 71
establishment as Commonwealth,
70
Racism
contribution of sociology to, 28

Racism (Cont.)
toward immigrants, 27-29
Rat allowances, 2
Rats
carriers of bubonic plague, 1
control programs, 2
danger to children, 2-4
environmental hazard to poor, 1-3
health hazard to Puerto Ricans, 77
increased concentration by slum
clearance, 4
in individual homes, 2
lack of governmental concern, 1-3
in large buildings, 2

Schizophrenia
causes, 132
relation to poverty, 129-30
School lunch programs, 126
Segregation. See Black Americans,
segregation
Settlement house movement, 34-35
"Ship fever," 31
Simkins v. Moses H. Cone Memorial
Hospital, 161
Sit-in demonstrations, 46
Slavery, 39-44
emancipation from, 42-43
in Europe, 40-41
impact on black Americans, 41-42
slave trade, 39-40
abolition, 40
mortality rate, 39
role of West Indies, 40
survival traits, 42
Slum housing
conditions, 3-4
in New York City in 1858, 33
of 19th-century immigrants, 32-33
overcrowding, 4
rats, 2-4
Snyder Act, 95-96
Socioeconomic status. See also Poverty
and alcoholism, 142-43
correlation with intelligence, 136
and dental care, 58-59
and drug addiction, 143

Socioeconomic status (Cont.)
  and family planning, 57
  and health, 7-12, 49-51
  and health care, 10-11, 148-49
  of health professionals, 147-51
  and infant mortality rates, 8-10
  and life expectancy, 8
  and maternal mortality rates, 8, 58
  and mental development, 137-38
    negative self-image, 138
    preschool experiences, 137
    teacher expectations, 137-38
  and mental health, 7-8, 129-44
  and mental illness. See Mental illness and socioeconomic status
  and premature birth, 123
  and preventive health care, 54
  and suicide, 141-42
Spanish-American War, 70
Spanish-speaking minorities. See Cubans; Mexican-Americans; Puerto Ricans
Starr, Ellen Gates, 34
Strauss, Nathan, 34
Suicide
  among black Americans, 142
  geographic distribution, 142
  among Mexican-Americans, 142
  among native Americans, 100, 101

Suicide (Cont.)
  and other self-destructive behaviours, 142-43
  and socioeconomic status, 141-42
Susto, 84

Trachoma, 97-98
Treaty of Guadalupe Hidalgo, 64
Tuberculosis
  lack of public support for research and therapy, 15
  among native Americans, 101-4
    among Navaho, 103-4
    control tests of Isoniazid, 103-4
    incidence, 103
    mortality rate, 101
  among Puerto Rican in United States, 77-78
  in Puerto Rico, 77
  socioeconomic distribution, 15

Universal Negro Improvement Association, 45

Wald, Lillian, 34, 35
Washington, Booker T., 44, 45
Wheeler Howard Act, 96